ACHIEVING
Your Personal
Health GOALS

A Patient's Guide

ACHIEVING
Your Personal Health GOALS
A Patient's Guide

JAMES W. MOLD, MD, MPH

Full Court Press

For permission requests, please address
Full Court Press
1001 Blackwood Mountain Rd
Chapel Hill, NC 27516

Published 2017 by Full Court Press
Printed in the United States of America

19 18 17   1 2 3 4

ISBN 978-0-692-92623-9 (paperback)
ISBN 978-0-692-92624-6 (eBook)

Library of Congress Control Number: 2017953080

Table of Contents

Preface

"The Doctor we have in mind, then, is no longer a general practitioner and by no means always a family practitioner. His essential characteristic, surely, is that he is looking after people as people and not as problems."

—*T.F. Fox*

Our Ailing Health Care System

Our health care system faces major challenges. Health care costs continue to increase. News reports heralding the soaring price tag and the impact of health care costs on American businesses are as common as reports of melting glaciers or trouble in the Middle East. And as the number of diagnostic and treatment options increase in parallel with rising expectations, it is hard to know what to do about it. Development of guidelines to standardize care, implementation of electronic record systems to increase efficiency, incentives for doctors and patients to reduce costs, and various forms of rationing (i.e., limiting access to high-cost tests and treatments based upon insurance coverage, age, or urgency) are all being tried. Free market enthusiasts advocate for greater transparency in quality and costs and higher insurance co-pays so that patients can force quality up and costs down.

At the same time, lower cost strategies like delivery of preventive services continue to be underutilized. Fewer than half of cigarette smokers report having been advised by their doctors to stop smoking. Only half of those with elevated blood pressure have their blood pressure under control. Nearly half of adults between 50 and 75 years of age have not been screened within 10 years for colon cancer, only 73% of women have had a mammogram within 2 years, and fewer than 75% of children have had all recommended immunizations by the age of 3.

Electronic medical records hold the promise of higher quality care at a lower cost. However, rather than enhancing communication between physicians and patients, computerization appears to have had the opposite effect, at least within the examination room.

Despite the rapidly increasing number of seniors in the American population, very few doctors choose to practice geriatrics, primarily because it is perceived to be too complicated and too time-consuming. Most physicians and a majority of their patients view aging as progressive decline rather than a continuing process of psychological and spiritual growth. Discussions about death and dying between health care professionals and their patients are infrequent and uncomfortable.

In a time of substantial access to medical information, people want to play a larger role in the health care decisions that affect them. Health care professionals have responded by becoming less paternalistic, but their patients remain dissatisfied. They want health care to be even more collaborative. "Shared decision-making" is the new buzzword, but something important still seems to be missing.

A Different Approach

What if things could be different? What if all of these challenges could be met not by additional payment reforms or new forms of rationing, and not by reorganizing services or by admonishing clinicians to spend more time listening to their patients?

What if all we need is a change in perspective, a different lens through which to view health and health care?

I'm convinced that such a shift in thinking is not only possible and desirable, but necessary, even critical.

I am also aware — and you should be forewarned — that while it will be easy for you to *understand* the changes I am proposing, they will not be easy to *implement*. This book is specifically *not* written for health care professionals who are likely to misunderstand, criticize, and downplay the importance of what I am suggesting. It is written for people like you who periodically rely on the health care system to achieve your health goals.

It is difficult to explain something new without contrasting it with the status quo. For that reason my description of modern medicine will at times sound highly critical. In fact, there are good reasons why our health care system has evolved the way it has, and tremendous progress has resulted from the current approach. However, every method eventually reaches the end of its utility, and I believe that in health care we have reached that point. I am not alone in this belief. Many doctors are dissatisfied with the way they are being forced to practice, but they don't know what to do about it.

Modern medicine arose in the 1800s during a time when biologists were busy classifying plants and animals, and physicians were correlating signs and symptoms with autopsy findings. It is therefore understandable that the focus of early clinicians was on the classification and correction of bodily abnormalities. Since then, doctors have become so good at this that we can now identify many abnormalities even before they begin to cause problems. And once symptoms develop, there is almost no limit to the number of tests that can be done to identify the cause. However, there is no clear method for deciding which symptoms *need to be* diagnosed or which abnormalities *need to be* corrected.

If you see a doctor and want to be tested, diagnosed, and/or treated for a particular condition or conditions, you most likely will be. If multiple abnormalities are identified, you will probably be advised to address all or most of them. The assumption is that by correcting every abnormality, the desired outcomes, such as survival and a better quality of life, will result. Unfortunately, this indirect approach, which

I will call "problem-oriented" care, doesn't always result in the best outcomes for a variety of reasons, and it is very, very expensive and sometimes even dangerous.

What if instead we took a *direct* approach? What if, before deciding whether diagnosis, treatment, or any other particular strategy, was warranted, we first agreed upon the desired outcomes (goals) and let *those* direct our actions? Would such a *goal-directed* approach help us do a better job of deciding which tests and treatments are worth doing? And could such an approach result in more person-centered care, better outcomes, and lower health care costs?

In this book I will argue that it could and would.

Let's look at a simple example: Jeremy was a 33-year-old engineer who, at the insistence of his wife, made an appointment with her primary care doctor to discuss a shoulder problem he'd had for more than a decade. The problem began with a high school sports injury. Jeremy had been a very good baseball pitcher, but his sports career had been cut short because of the injury to his shoulder. Since high school, he had continued to endure intermittent pain, which had prompted him to see various health professionals over the years, including several primary care doctors, an orthopedic surgeon, and a physical therapist. Jeremy had tried periods of rest, heat, and ice, a variety of exercises, an injection, and anti-inflammatory medications, each of which only helped temporarily. The orthopedist had offered to perform surgery, but had also said that he couldn't guarantee the shoulder would be significantly better afterward.

Jeremy's new primary care doctor took a different approach. He began by asking Jeremy, "How does the pain affect your life? What does it keep you from doing?" After considering these questions, Jeremy reported that the most important thing he was unable to do was to hunt deer with a bow and arrow, a hobby he had acquired as a teenager and had shared with his father and brother prior to the shoulder problem. At that moment, an imaginary light bulb appeared to switch on in Jeremy's mind. "You know, I've seen some deer hunters using crossbows," he said. "I could probably do that, but to get a crossbow license I think I would need a doctor's note saying that I am unable to use a traditional bow."

His doctor wrote the note, and soon Jeremy was enjoying hunting again.

Jeremy's case provides a simple introduction to the concepts discussed in this book. His doctor essentially flipped the script—instead of attempting to diagnose Jeremy's *problem* and offering ways to correct the abnormality (a torn rotator cuff), he helped Jeremy identify his *personal health goals*. This led to a simple (and in this case non-medical) strategy, and an immediate improvement in quality of life.

I've written this book because I believe that the goal-directed approach that Jeremy's primary care doctor employed is key to the future of health care … that focusing on a patient's goals is perhaps the simplest and best way to reduce soaring medical bills and truly improve the lives of people of all ages.

My Personal Journey

Many of the ideas discussed in this book arose from my clinical experiences providing care for people over the age of 75. Health care professionals who focus on the care of the elderly know how poorly our health care system handles individuals with multiple physical impairments in combination with social, environmental, and financial challenges. Care for the elderly is often inadequate (e.g., a lack of attention to basic functional and social needs), excessive (too many referrals, tests, procedures, and medications), poorly coordinated, and incredibly expensive. The failure of the health care system to meet the needs of the elderly should be viewed as a societal warning signal, like the canary in the coal mine.

There have been other warnings. Decades ago, women said they no longer wanted pregnancy to be treated like a problem, and, through their efforts, obstetrical care became more humane. The field of Sports Medicine arose because athletes needed a different approach to care. And the hospice movement resulted from the inability of the health care system to adequately address the needs of those in the process of dying.

I decided to become a family doctor in 1973 after spending time with several small-town family doctors during medical school. The new specialty of Family Medicine, intended to elevate the status and effectiveness of "old-time" general practice by adding additional scientific training, had been established four years earlier. In those early days, many of us who chose to enter the field were, in some ways, revolutionaries. Children of the sixties, we were convinced we could make health care more humane. Of course, we weren't the first to raise concerns about the direction health care seemed to be headed. Francis Peabody, alarmed by the trends he was seeing in medical education, published a paper in the 1927 Journal of the American Medical Association, in which he felt compelled to state the obvious, that "…the secret of the care of the patient is caring for the patient."

After six years in private practice in a small town in North Carolina, I joined the faculty of an academic department of Family Medicine. I had lofty goals. I intended to change the way doctors were trained. But I had underestimated the challenge. While I may have had a positive influence on students during introductory courses in clinical care, the effects were subsequently buried beneath an avalanche of problem-oriented content.

By the mid-1980's, the revolutionary spirit that had attracted me to Family Medicine was rapidly waning. The push for acceptance of Family Medicine within academia had swept away all hope of fusing medical science with the personal care provided by general practitioners. Most medical training in the United States was and still is controlled by subspecialists, who are, by definition of their disciplines, disease-oriented. Their emphasis on the science of diseases had continued to both fragment and depersonalize care.

During that time, however, a new group of revolutionaries began to emerge: The field of geriatrics was born in England and was spreading to the United States. I quickly joined them and spent the next decade developing geriatric clinical and teaching services at the University of Oklahoma Health Sciences Center, and in the surrounding community. During that time I learned to work collaboratively with other health care professionals, nurses, occupational, physical and speech therapists, social workers, mental health professionals, dentists, pharmacists, and others. In geriatrics, teamwork was valued.

I also began to give lectures on the care of older people. Interestingly, the topic most often requested was "Normal Aging Changes." After giving that talk dozens of times, I began to wonder why it was so important to doctors to be able to differentiate between the physical changes associated with "normal" aging from those resulting from factors like diseases, exposures, and injuries.

Finally it dawned on me. The problem-oriented approach to health care can only be applied when "normal" and "abnormal" are clearly distinguished. But for me, that distinction didn't seem to be that important. It seemed to me that the goal of medicine should be to help people live longer and enjoy life more, regardless of the cause of their symptoms. For example, just because menopause is part of "normal aging," it doesn't mean we should ignore the resulting symptoms if those symptoms are reducing quality of life.

My understanding of the differences between problem-oriented and goal-directed care became clearer while taking care of patients at an inpatient geriatric rehabilitation unit, where most patients were recovering from a stroke, amputation, or hip fracture. On this unit, I met each week with a case manager, a social worker, a nurse, a physical therapist, an occupational therapist, and a speech therapist, all caring for the same set of patients. The purpose of these team conferences was ostensibly to establish patients' goals and to document progress.

I remember thinking, "What a great idea!"— only to be quickly disappointed that there was so little dialogue at these conferences, and virtually no patient involvement. The case manager would ask each team member what *their* goals were for the patient, what progress had been made to date, and what their plans were for the week. There was almost no back-and-forth discussion. I remember wondering whose goals we were documenting, and why we weren't all working toward the same ones.

I also remember visiting the Activities of Daily Living room on this unit, where patients worked on basic skills like eating, bathing, dressing, etc. Seeing one of my patients who had experienced a stroke sitting in front of the stove learning to cook one-handed, I said, "I didn't know you liked to cook." "I don't," he said. "So why are you learning to cook one-handed?" I asked. "I have no idea," he said. "The therapist told me I needed to do this." Evidently, a functional evaluation had identified that this patient was unable to cook, and so the "goal" was to solve that problem.

After reading this book, some may worry that I am throwing out the baby (medical science) with the bathwater (depersonalized care)… that goal-directed care is soft, less rigorous, and/or that by not addressing every abnormality, something important might be missed. Please understand—I am not proposing that individuals like Jeremy should *never* have a shoulder operation. All I am suggesting is that the strategies proposed and considered should be directly related to the patient's goals. Focusing on goals simply provides a more humane framework within which to apply modern medical science. It focuses the attention of the health care system on patients rather than their diseases.

I am confident that the health care system will evolve over time to become more goal-directed. It will because it has to, if for no other reason than that we can no longer afford to identify and fix every abnormality.

How to Read This Book

In Section 1, I will explain how a goal-directed approach could improve four key health outcomes and how it would differ from the current problem-oriented approach. In Section 2, the focus will shift to the obstacles that would have to be overcome if goal-directed care is to be implemented by the health care system. While some of you may be tempted to skip this somewhat depressing section, I included it because I think you will need the information in it to make the system work to your advantage. Finally, in Section 3, I will describe how understanding the principles of goal-directed care can improve the help you and your family members receive even before the system adopts them. In the final two chapters I have tried to provide very specific suggestions about how you can help your doctors provide you with goal-directed care.

The cases (like Jeremy's) cited throughout the book are, unless otherwise stated, drawn from my 36 years of experience as a family physician. Patient names have, of course, been changed. Jeremy's case involved improving quality of life, one of the four health care goals I will discuss. The other three goals are prevention of premature death and disability, facilitation of optimal growth and development, and increasing the likelihood of a comfortable and respectful death. Under certain circumstances, other goals may come into play, such as protecting the life of a fetus or reducing a caregiver's burden, but the principles involved are similar. In each case, the idea is to focus on the goals before deciding on what, if anything, to do.

Let's begin.

SECTION 1:
The Goals of Health and Health Care

"The kind of health that men desire most is not necessarily a state in which they experience physical vigor and a sense of well-being, not even one giving them long life. It is, instead, the condition best suited to reach goals that each individual formulates for himself."

—*Rene' Dubos, 1959*

"Health is a complete state of physical, mental and social well-being, and not merely the absence of disease or infirmity."

—*World Health Organization*

Medical care in the United States and most other developed countries is still firmly rooted in the idea that "health" is defined by the absence of disease. This problem-oriented definition and approach to care is based upon the assumption that correcting all of your abnormalities (i.e., curing your diseases and other defects) will result in a longer and more pleasant life. And if you suffer from only one or a few easily-correctable problems, that assumption generally holds true.

However, we doctors have become so good at identifying abnormalities that very few people have only a few of them, and most are not so easily corrected. When my 22-year-old otherwise very healthy brother saw a subspecialist for a lump on his thyroid gland, he glanced over at his medical record and saw that there were eight problems listed on his problem list.

Most ordinary people think of health differently. I suspect that most of us view life as a journey characterized by amazing opportunities and tremendous challenges. Had we not been taught to think otherwise, we would probably define health as the ability to derive the greatest possible value from the trip. The things we value most include *being able to do the things we find meaningful and enjoyable for as long as we can; meeting, overcoming, and learning from the challenges along the way; and then dying peacefully having had the opportunity to reach our full potential as human beings.*

This very reasonable definition of "health" suggests that our four major goals are, and the goals of the health care we receive should therefore be: 1) prevention of premature death and disability; 2) maintenance or improvement of quality of life; 3) preparation for a good death; and 4) maximization of personal growth and development.

The premise of this book is that shifting the focus of health care from problem solving to attainment of those four goals will improve the outcomes that matter to people, while avoiding unnecessary testing and treatments, reducing health care costs, and enhancing collaboration between doctors and their patients.

It might be hard to believe, but this simple premise, which I'm guessing seems rather obvious to many of you, is in fact a very radical proposition.

In this section of the book, I will explain how a goal-directed approach would lead to different strategies and result in better outcomes. When I am critical of problem-oriented care, health care professionals, or the modern health care system, it is simply to provide a clear contrast between problem-oriented and goal-directed care. In many situations the problem-oriented approach still works well, but we can, and must, do better. The goal-directed approach described here is a way to make health care better.

CHAPTER 1:

Prevention of Premature Death and Disability

"You have two lives. The second one begins when you realize you only have one."

—Confucius

"As long as you are breathing there is more right with you than wrong with you."

—Jon Kabat-Zinn

Changing the Focus

I often use the following fictional case to introduce goal-directed health care to physicians.

Mr. Sawyer is an 68-year-old retired welder. A widower, he lives in an apartment by himself. He requires supplemental oxygen 24 hours a day because of emphysema. However, Mr. Sawyer still enjoys his somewhat limited life, which includes reading, television, e-mailing friends, and going out to eat twice a week at a cafeteria close to his apartment. His two children and four grandchildren visit him nearly every week. He quit smoking several years ago, has had the influenza and pneumonia vaccinations, and is using the inhalers that his doctor recommended for his emphysema.

One of Mr. Sawyer's primary goals is, quite simply, staying alive. If you were his doctor, what strategies might you recommend to him that could extend his life?

When presented with this case, most doctors draw a blank. Or they repeat the things that Mr. Sawyer has done or is doing (e.g., smoking cessation, immunizations and inhalers). When I ask them what illness will most likely end Mr. Sawyer's life, they correctly say lung failure, most likely triggered by an infection (bronchitis or pneumonia). But when I ask them what then could be done to prevent a lung infection, they struggle.

Next, I ask where the germs that cause lung infections are likely to come from. Most answer that viruses are likely to come from contact with others who are infected, and some go on to say that Mr. Sawyer should be advised to avoid close contact with people with coughs or congestion. They may or may not recall that Mr. Sawyer has children and grandchildren who visit him regularly, and in the many years I've been spinning this hypothetical tale, no doctor has so far suggested that Mr. Sawyer tell his family to stay away when they have an infection or advising Mr. Sawyer to wash his hands after going through the cafeteria line before touching his nose or eyes.

For Mr. Sawyer, these simple measures would not only be helpful. They could be life saving.

Finally I ask the doctors where the bacteria might come from that could cause the more serious types of pneumonia. Most of them haven't really ever thought about it. As it turns out, the bacteria that cause pneumonia usually come from the mouth, and particularly from around the teeth. In fact, at least one well-designed study found that regular dental hygiene significantly reduced the risk of pneumonia among a group of nursing home residents. Thus, advising Mr. Sawyer to brush his teeth regularly and to see a dental hygienist every six months could be beneficial. There is also evidence suggesting that certain medicines that reduce stomach acid may increase the risk of pneumonia in people with chronic lung disease, so Mr. Sawyer should be warned to avoid those over-the-counter medications.

Brush your teeth, avoid sick people, wash your hands after contact with potentially contaminated surfaces, avoid a few specific medications … all very simple steps that Mr. Sawyer's doctors should be recommending.

But most of the doctors I talk to about Mr. Sawyer are left scratching their heads.

There are many reasons for this. One is that doctors have been taught to think that diseases have single causes. For example, the cause of bacterial pneumonia is understood to be a specific bacterium (germ). Therefore, for most doctors, the treatment for bacterial pneumonia is to kill the germ with antibiotics. The truth is much more complex. Most health challenges are the result of a combination of factors. To get bacterial pneumonia, lots of the right kind of germ must first be present in the individual's mouth, nose, or throat. Poor oral hygiene, weakened resistance, dentures, or certain medicines that reduce saliva production can promote bacterial growth. The bacteria must then travel to the lungs and fail to be cleared by mucous production and coughing. Lastly, the body's defense system must fail to keep the bacteria from multiplying and invading the lung tissue.

Addressing *any* of these factors could potentially prevent the development of bacterial pneumonia. And giving antibiotics alone may not be sufficient to cure the problem.

In addition to the strategies already mentioned, Mr. Sawyer's doctor might consider recommending sugar-free lemon drops to increase saliva production or artificial saliva, since Mr. Sawyer's mouth is likely to be somewhat dry from his inhalers. A well-balanced diet and possibly a daily multivitamin could insure that he is getting the vitamins and minerals needed for his immune system to function well. Medicines in the ACE inhibitor class (e.g., lisinopril or ramipril) might increase his cough reflex, helping him clear bacteria before it enters his lungs, though this has only been studied in stroke patients. Sources of chronic emotional stress and sleep problems, which might reduce immune function, could also be addressed. While the effectiveness of some of these strategies can certainly be debated, they are nonetheless reasonable to consider, simple to implement, and unlikely to cause harm.

Why do doctors have such difficulty with a case like Mr. Sawyer's? Why don't they think of simple, well-known, preventive strategies, like avoidance of sick children and hand washing after touching public counter tops? And why don't doctors consider dental hygiene and avoidance of acid blocking medicines?

The surprising answer to these questions is that most doctors are not accustomed to thinking about their patients' individual health goals. Their assumption is that successful treatment of a person's diseases will result in a longer and more pleasant life.

In other words, they approach health and health care *indirectly*: focusing on the disease rather than on the goal - in this case survival. And because they haven't practiced goal-directed thinking, they have trouble doing it.

Prevention

Most people, if asked, say they would like to avoid a *premature* death (i.e. dying from something that could have been prevented). They would also prefer not to become disabled. For the most part, the same strategies used to prevent premature death also prevent or delay disability, so for all practical purposes, these two important health goals—the prevention of both premature death and premature disability—can be considered together. For example, prevention of a stroke by reducing blood pressure can both delay death and prevent one cause of disability.

Doctors are taught to think about three types of prevention: primary, secondary, and tertiary. It will be useful for you to have a working understanding of these terms.

Primary prevention is defined as implementing a preventive health measure before a problem has developed. Examples include eating a healthy diet, being physically active, getting sufficient sleep, and getting recommended immunizations. It also includes avoiding hazardous substances such as tobacco and the consumption of too much alcohol, and reducing the risk of injuries by wearing seatbelts and wearing a helmet when riding a bicycle or motorcycle. Some medicines can also prevent the development of future health problems. For example, taking low-dose aspirin can prevent heart attacks, strokes, and colon cancer in those at risk for these conditions. In general, the payoffs for engaging in primary prevention are significant, and the risks are small.

Secondary prevention involves finding potential health challenges after they have developed but before they have begun to cause symptoms. This form of prevention is usually called "screening." Pap smears to detect cervical cancer, mammograms to detect breast cancer, colonoscopies to find colon cancer, blood tests for prostate cancer, and CT scans to find early lung cancers are all examples of secondary prevention or screening. So are measurements of blood pressure, blood sugar, and cholesterol. The assumption is that, by discovering the condition and/or detecting risk earlier, treatment will be more effective.

Compared to primary prevention, secondary prevention generally results in smaller increases in life expectancy, and the benefits tend to accrue somewhat farther in the future. For example, it takes about 10 years, on average, for someone to benefit from colon cancer screening, whereas a flu shot protects within 6 weeks and aspirin reduces the risk of heart attacks in men and strokes in women shortly after the first dose. And because no screening test is perfectly accurate, some people who are screened end up having unnecessary follow-up tests and treatments because of false positive test results.

Tertiary prevention involves the treatment of already present, symptomatic conditions to prevent those conditions from causing premature death or disability. As a general rule, tertiary prevention is the least effective and most expensive type of prevention. However, because tertiary prevention involves treating known medical conditions with established medical tests and prescription medicines, it is the type of prevention most consistently provided by doctors. In fact, most doctors don't ordinarily think of it as prevention at all. They call it "treatment of disease" or "disease management." For example, treating cancer with chemotherapy is a form of tertiary prevention, because its goal is to prevent premature death (i.e. to extend life). Another example is the treatment of people with known coronary artery disease with a statin (a type of cholesterol-lowering medicine) to prevent heart attacks.

Prioritizing Primary Prevention – Doing What's Most Important

Most of you can probably think of a long list of things you should be doing to reduce your risk of premature death or disability. For many people, this list of *shoulds* is so long it is overwhelming, and so they don't end up doing anything. "Everybody has to die of something, right?" is a common refrain.

But there's good news. Simply doing the most effective three or four things on your list will often produce nearly the same benefit as doing everything. This is called the law of diminishing returns. Because each thing you do reduces your risk somewhat, each time you do something effective you reduce the benefit that can be obtained from subsequent strategies.

If it isn't clear yet which health challenges are likely to cause your death (unlike Mr. Sawyer), you will have to take a very broad approach. Since primary prevention is usually more effective than secondary and tertiary prevention, it is generally wise to focus on primary preventive measures first. The choice of strategies depends a great deal on your personal risk profile. For example, if you smoke cigarettes, you can gain more additional life, on average, from quitting smoking than from nearly any other preventive measure. Or if you are a young, African American male living in an unsafe neighborhood in Chicago, you will benefit most from strategies that reduce your risk of physical injury, addiction, and incarceration. For those addicted to alcohol, alcoholism treatment will have a far greater impact on life expectancy than all other preventive strategies combined.

While the problem-oriented approach suggests that you should address *every* risk factor and apply *every* available preventive measure recommended for you, a goal-directed approach suggests that you focus first on the measures most likely to provide the greatest benefit to you, given your personal risk profile and your abilities and preferences. Then, you can decide if it is worth it to do the rest.

Changing the Conversation: Investing in Your Health

Mrs. Gooch, a 57 year-old African American mother of three and grandmother of 6, had been a patient of mine for more than 10 years. Her medical diagnoses included diabetes, high blood pressure, and arthritis. During one of her office visits I said to her, "You still seem to be enjoying life a lot." She replied that she was. I said, "I assume that one of the reasons you come to see me is so I can help you stay alive as long as possible." Again she said, "Yes." Then I asked her, "What kinds of things would you still like to see and do before you die?"

She began to talk about her grandchildren, about family gatherings, graduations and marriages. I asked, "What do you think would be the *most* important thing you could do, with my help, which could increase the chance that you will live to see those things happen?" She said, "I should probably stop smoking." When I agreed, she said, "I'm going to do it." And she did.

Encouraging Mrs. Gooch to focus on her goal caused her to become invested in the strategies to achieve it. By "invested,"

I mean simply that Mrs. Gooch saw maximizing time with her family as important enough to make a significant investment of time and energy to extend her life.

In the current problem-oriented framework smoking would have been identified as one of Mrs. Gooch's problems, and she would have been advised to quit. The difference between a goal-directed approach and a problem-oriented one may seem subtle, but, in my experience, it is huge. A goal-directed approach ties the strategy - smoking cessation, to a meaningful personal goal - survival, and a set of objectives - valued life events. It frames the issue in positive (i.e., goal achievement) rather than negative (i.e., correcting an abnormality) terms. The positive approach is almost always more effective because it encourages patients to make a greater investment in their health. And greater investment almost *always* leads to greater returns.

Doing Only What is Necessary

A goal-directed approach would reduce the use of tests and treatments that are unrelated to your goals.

A close friend, Dora Menninger, celebrated her 101th birthday this past year. However, a few months after her 100th birthday she began to have trouble getting out of bed. She was unable to make her legs work properly. At that time, Dora was living in her own home, completely independent. She was able to call her daughter, who took her to the local hospital emergency room.

For several years Dora had been treated for lumbar spinal stenosis, a condition in which overgrowth of bone in the lower spine cause pressure on the spinal cord, which can eventually result in paralysis. Since no other cause was found on initial testing at the hospital, the spinal stenosis was believed to be the most likely cause of her leg trouble. However, since she needed additional X-rays and a neurosurgical evaluation and because she was now unable to care for herself, she was admitted to the hospital.

On admission to the hospital Dora's blood pressure was elevated, so she was given medication to lower it. Unfortunately the medicine caused a significant drop in her blood pressure that reduced the amount of blood reaching a vulnerable area of her brain. The result was a stroke, which left Dora paralyzed on one side of her body and unable to speak. After months of physical, occupational, and speech therapy, Dora now lives in an assisted living center.

You are probably wondering how important it was to lower Dora's blood pressure. The answer is that *it was not important at all*, since blood pressure reduction was completely unrelated to any of Dora's goals.

So why did her doctor do it? The answer requires a brief discussion of blood pressure. Bear with me. Because so many of us will be told we have high blood pressure at some point in our lives, this is important!

If someone were to measure the blood pressure of every adult in the United States, the results would fit nicely on a bell-shaped curve. Most people would have blood pressures between 100/70 and 160/100. A few would have blood pressures higher or lower than that, but the vast majority would fall within that middle range.

Over a period of years, pressure on the inner walls of the heart and blood vessels can, in combination with other factors like smoking and high cholesterol levels, cause damage, which can eventually increase the risk of heart attacks, strokes, heart and kidney failure, and decreased circulation to the feet and legs. In other words, your pipes (blood vessels), pump (heart), and filter (kidneys) can wear out sooner when exposed to higher pressures over long periods of time. The higher the blood pressure and the longer it is elevated, the more likely it is that damage and unwanted consequences will occur.

So the bottom line is that the lower your blood pressure is, the longer your arteries, heart, and kidneys will last. The problem is that a certain amount of pressure is necessary to keep your blood flowing. That is why when your blood pressure is lowered too far, you feel lightheaded and weak, and you could experience serious harm, as in Mrs. Menninger's case.

Using the logic of problem-oriented care, a person with several blood pressure measurements above 140/90 is said to have "hypertension," the medical term for high blood pressure, while those with pressures of 139/89 or lower are said to be "normotensive" (normal). This somewhat arbitrary dividing line has been established by panels of experts based upon a balance of risks and benefits determined by clinical research. It is the line, required for problem-oriented care, which separates normal from abnormal. Once your average blood pressure is above 140/90, the focus becomes the problem/disease: hypertension. Mrs. Menninger's blood pressure was high; therefore, she was given medicine to lower it.

Clearly, there's something wrong here. In Mrs. Menninger's case, a goal-directed approach would have led her doctor to conclude that her blood pressure elevation was completely irrelevant. At the age of 100 with no evidence of serious heart or kidney disease or risk of bleeding, her life expectancy was too short for her to benefit from blood pressure reduction. (Remember, blood pressure elevation requires many years to cause harm.)

Like hypertension, many other "diseases" are defined by a line drawn through a bell-shaped curve. For example, diabetes is diagnosed when the before-meal (fasting) blood sugar levels are above 126. Until recently, that dividing line was 140. Lowering it to 126 has probably made no difference in the outcomes that matter to people with diabetes, but it has definitely increased the profits of pharmaceutical companies. Notice the number of advertisements for diabetes medicines.

"High cholesterol" is often diagnosed when the total cholesterol level is above 200 or the low density ("bad") cholesterol level is above 130. Depression is defined as the presence of feelings of sadness or loss of interest in usual activities for more than two weeks duration (Why not one week or three weeks?) plus at least 4 other symptoms from a list of 7 (Why not 3 or 5?)

The problem-oriented approach requires clear lines of separation between normal and abnormal. The context and personal circumstances diminish in importance once a diagnosis has been made. Each diagnostic label is linked to a treatment, often a medication.

Of course I am exaggerating to make a point. Experienced clinicians who know and care about their patients are able to balance the problem-oriented approach they were taught with an understanding of what is best for individual patients. However, there is no question that problem-oriented thinking can result in both over- and under-diagnosis and treatment simply because it fails to account for context and is disconnected from patients' goals.

When Survival is No Longer a Goal: Length versus Quality of Life

While staying alive is an important goal for most people, most of us can think of conditions under which death would be a blessing. Over a ten-year period, my partners and I asked every new patient seen in our geriatric practice to state which was more important to them: length of life or quality of life. Nearly all of our patients were over 65 years old; their average age was 78.

Eighty-two percent said quality of life.

When we took a deeper look at their answers, we found something interesting: Those who chose "length of life" over "quality of life" were more likely to be disabled.

That surprised us. It seemed counterintuitive. Why would people with disabilities be more likely to want to stay alive? In fact the same phenomenon has been noted in other studies, some of which have surveyed the same people over time. The most likely explanation is that when we are doing well, we can't imagine being able to enjoy life with a serious disability. However, when disabilities inevitably occur, we discover that we can tolerate them much better than we thought we could, and we are reminded that life is precious and almost always better than the alternative.

We also asked patients, "What conditions, if permanent, would you consider to be worse than death?" We gave them a list of the options (shown in the table below). Initially many patients said that all of the conditions on the list would be worse than death. However, their answers changed when we put the question another way: "If you were in that condition and it was going to be permanent, and you then developed pneumonia, would you want us to give you antibiotics to treat the pneumonia?"

The proportion of people choosing each condition under those conditions is shown below:

CONDITION	PERCENTAGE OF PATIENTS SAYING THE CONDITION WOULD BE WORSE THAN DEATH
Unable to live alone	6%
Living in a nursing home	15%
Unable to make decisions for self	21%

CONDITION	PERCENTAGE OF PATIENTS SAYING THE CONDITION WOULD BE WORSE THAN DEATH
Painful terminal illness	36%
Unable to recognize family members	40%
Permanent coma	85%

Amazingly, only 40% of people said that being too confused to recognize members of their own family would be worse than death. To us, that suggested that survival is almost always considered preferable to the alternative, and that prevention of premature death is the most important health-related goal for most people.

Interestingly, when we looked for personal characteristics that might predict patients' opinions about conditions worse than death, we couldn't find a single one. Age, race, marital status, educational attainment, religion, and income were all poor predictors. That means that, while survival is almost always a goal, the point at which it isn't must be determined in conversation with each person. And because people often change their minds, that conversation must be repeated periodically.

Once you are clear, in your own mind, about what conditions you would consider worse than death, make sure you communicate that information to everyone who might be involved when decisions have to be made, especially close family members and your doctors.

When I first met Mrs. Delaney, she was a 74-year-old Caucasian widowed woman who had been brought to see me by her daughter because of problems with her short-term memory. Testing revealed that Mrs. Delaney's short-term memory was starting to fail, but her judgment and decision-making abilities were still working well. (Note: In most forms of dementia, including Alzheimers Disease, short term memory is the first symptom to appear.) With her daughter present, Mrs. Delaney said she would not want to be kept alive if she was no longer able to recognize close family members.

Three years later, Mrs. Delaney's thinking had continued to deteriorate, and she required nursing home care. After being in the nursing home for about a year, she could no longer recognize her daughter, who had visited her daily throughout her stay. At that point her daughter reminded me of her mother's directive. Based upon her previous statement that she would rather be dead than to be kept alive in this condition, I advised the nursing home staff and the medical team that life prolongation was no longer a goal for Mrs. Delaney. I told the staff to stop measuring her blood pressure and discontinued her blood pressure medicines. However during a period of staff turnover, the order was overlooked, and the doctor on call restarted the medicines. Her daughter called me the next day to let me know what had happened. I stopped the medicines again and briefed the new nurse and the on-call team.

About three months after that episode I received another call from her daughter, which began with, "Why did you write orders for a pneumonia shot for my mother? Doesn't that directly contradict her stated preference?" While handling the mountains of paperwork that came across my desk each day, I had signed a number of routine pneumonia vaccination orders that week – hers included   without even thinking about it. I apologized. Mrs. Delaney died peacefully a couple of months later with her daughter by her side.

This true story illustrates both the importance of discussing your wishes with key family members and your doctors and the difficulty the health care system has when survival is no longer a goal.

Trade-Offs

While prevention of premature death and disability is an important goal for most people, quality of life is also important and quite often requires strategies that are in direct conflict with those I have been discussing.

A few years ago, blood tests showed that my cholesterol was elevated. My doctor suggested that I take a cholesterol-lowering medicine called a statin. Up to that point in my life I had avoided taking medicines. When I had a headache or a backache, I rested. My philosophy has always been that the human body, improved over millions of years of natural selection, is probably better at healing itself than the pharmaceutical companies are. As a doctor, I am also very aware of the potential, sometimes serious side effects of medications. Faced with the prospect of taking a cholesterol-lowering medicine daily for the rest of my life, I was hesitant.

So my response was to ask my doctor several additional questions. The conversation went something like this:

―――――――――

Me: I understand that taking a statin will reduce my risk of having a heart attack, but by how much? I mean, what is my risk if I don't take the drug and what would it be if I took it?

Doctor: I'm not sure, but I can look it up on my computer (see *http://www.cvriskcalculator.com/*)... The computer says that your risk of having a heart attack is about 12% over the next 10 years. But that estimate doesn't take into account the fact that your father had a heart attack at age 52, so it's probably a bit higher than that, perhaps 16%. Taking a statin would reduce your 10-year risk by about 25% to 12%.

Me: So, I could reduce my risk by about 4% from what it is now. OK. And if I did have a heart attack, what is the chance that it would kill me or leave me disabled?

Doctor: Well, if you got to the hospital quickly, the cardiologists are now very good at opening up the clogged artery. I'd guess that about 25% of heart attacks are still fatal, and another 25% cause the heart muscle to be significantly weakened, but those are just educated guesses.

Me: So, you're saying that if I take this medicine every

> day for ten years, I could lower my risk of death
> or disability by 2%?
>
> <u>Doctor</u>: Yes, but that is just one way to look at it. If
> you are in that 2% then you would have avoided
> dying needlessly or having a weakened heart.

What I didn't tell my doctor was that my greatest concern
about taking a statin was the possibility that it might cause
muscle weakness. This concern was based on one small study
I'd read that suggested that nearly everyone who takes a statin
has some degree of weakening of the leg muscles. While most
doctors would dispute the results of that one small study
(with good reasons), all of us have irrational fears and beliefs.
In my case, I was an aging weekend warrior still trying to
play pick-up basketball with much younger players.

It took me several months to decide to take the statin. I
still play basketball, and I can't say that the medicine has
affected my game. (I still can't jump.) Still, I'm glad that I
weighed the possible trade-offs of taking this medication
before deciding to take it.

Taking medications, following a special diet, having regular
medical check-ups or regular blood tests, or doing anything
else that you would prefer not to do in order to increase your
length of life, will reduce your quality of life to some degree.
It is therefore important that you discuss with your doctor
the size of the expected benefit, and the potential hazards and
costs, so that you can decide whether the negative effects on
your quality of life are worth the positive benefits on your
length of life.

WHAT GOAL-DIRECTED CARE WOULD LOOK LIKE – PART 1

1. Your primary health care team would make a special effort to learn about you *as a human being*, documenting that information on the opening page of your health record. Additional information would be added over time. Your personal profile would be the first thing your health care providers would see when they opened your record.

2. Each year you would be encouraged to go online or come to the office to fill out a comprehensive health risk assessment, followed by a discussion of your current life situation and goals. Based upon your risk profile, a computer program would produce a list of preventive strategies you could consider, including how much you could expect to benefit from each strategy. You would then develop or update a plan for the coming year with strategies to prevent premature death and disability consistent with your values, preferences, resources, and limitations. It would include reminders and encouragement throughout the year, as well as an expectation that the strategies might need to be adjusted.

3. As new health challenges or risk factors arose, you and your primary care team would discuss their potential impact on length of life and risk of future disabilities, and your wellness plan would be adjusted accordingly.

4. Your progress would be monitored by plotting your estimated life expectancy — the number of years you were predicted to live — given your age, gender, race, risk factors, and the measures you had taken to prevent premature death — as well as health expectancy — the number of years you are predicted to live free from a significant disability.

5. The annual review of risk factors and goals would include a discussion of conditions that you would consider to be worse than death.

CHAPTER 2:
Quality of Life

"The quality of life is determined by its activities."

—*Aristotle*

When Ziggy asked the wise man on the hill, "What is the meaning of life?"

The wise man's answer was, "Doing stuff."

—*From a Ziggy cartoon by Tom Wilson*

Enjoying Life

Quality of life is the issue of greatest concern for most people who don't yet have a life-threatening illness. While quality of life is a broad concept that includes more than just health, health certainly plays a major role in one's ability to enjoy life. Even within the health domain, there are several aspects of quality of life that could be considered. In this chapter I will focus primarily on one of these, the ability to participate in essential and meaningful life activities. I am defining "essential activities" as those activities required to function on a day-to-day basis in ones chosen setting, and "meaningful life activities" as activities that give life value, meaning, and purpose.

Essential Activities

Mrs. Palmer was an 80-year-old retired school teacher who lived independently in her own home. I became her primary care doctor when her previous doctor moved out of state. He had been evaluating her for weight loss and some abnormal liver tests. As part of my usual approach, I asked her to tell me about a typical day in her life.

She said, "I get up quite early, around 6AM, go into the bathroom, wash myself off with a washcloth, and then get dressed. Then I spend the next hour or so getting my socks and shoes on." Of course, I stopped her at that point and asked her why on earth it took so long to put on her socks and shoes. She said that arthritis in her hips and knees made it hard to bend far enough forward to reach her feet without stretching, bouncing, and struggling.

Because of my experience in a rehabilitation setting, I knew enough to refer Mrs. Palmer to an occupational therapist, who, in one 45 minute session, taught her how to use a sock donner and a long-handled shoe horn. With those two inexpensive pieces of equipment, she was able to dress in about five minutes.

The problem-oriented approach to Mrs. Palmer's arthritis would probably have unfolded in one of the following ways. Since she was not complaining of pain, it might not have been addressed at all or, based upon physical examination findings, it might have been listed on the problem list in her medical record. If she had mentioned stiffness or trouble walking, her doctor might have ordered X-rays and lab tests, which would have confirmed the diagnosis of osteoarthritis. Management might have included Tylenol or an anti-inflammatory medication, injections, and potentially referral to an orthopedic surgeon, measures which would probably not have substantially improved Mrs. Palmer's daily life.

Tragically Mrs. Palmer was, in fact, talked into knee replacement surgery several years later by a family member. Because of post-operative complications, she ended up losing most of her leg.

Meaningful Activities

Let's consider another example.

When I met Mr. Washington, he had been admitted to the hospital three times already that year for congestive heart failure, a condition in which the heart muscle is too weak to keep up with the needs of the body. The doctors-in-training under my supervision had correctly determined that the reason for the hospitalizations was that Mr. Washington did not always take his heart medicines, medicines required to keep fluid from building up in his legs and lungs. However, they had been unable to figure out why. One of them even speculated that he liked being in the hospital, a theory which Mr. Washington steadfastly denied.

I found Mr. Washington to be a very pleasant, if reserved, man with at least average intelligence. He had no trouble engaging with me or answering my questions. Our conversation went something like this:

***

> <u>Me</u>: I understand that you have had this same trouble before with fluid buildup. The other doctors who have seen you think it is because you don't always take your heart medicines.
>
> <u>Mr. Washington</u>: Yes, sir. I suspect that's right.
>
> <u>Me</u>: Can you help me understand why that happens?
>
> <u>Mr. Washington</u>: OK. What can I tell you?
>
> <u>Me</u>: Why don't you start by telling me where you live and what a typical day is like for you?
>
> <u>Mr. Washington</u>: Well, I live on the eighth floor of a high-rise apartment building about five blocks from here. I generally get up and take a shower, then get dressed and have a little breakfast. There's a senior citizen's center on the first floor. I generally go down and spend the morning there playing dominoes or checkers. You know. They serve lunch and have some kind of program. Then I go up to my apartment, take a nap, watch TV or read

the paper, fix my supper, watch some TV and go to bed.

<u>Me</u>: So why don't you always take your heart medicines?

<u>Mr. Washington</u>: Well, you see, there's not but one bathroom at the senior center and lots of people in line to use it. When I take the heart medicine, I have to pee a lot, and when I have to go, it can't wait, so sometimes I decide not to take it.

<u>Me</u>: So why don't you take the medicine in the afternoon, after you get back to your apartment?

<u>Mr. Washington</u>: The doctors told me I had to take it first thing in the morning.

<u>Me</u>: That was just so you wouldn't have to get up in the night to pee.

<u>Mr. Washington</u>: Getting up in the night wouldn't be no problem for me.

<u>Me</u>: Then you could start taking all of your heart medicines when you get back up to your apartment after visiting the senior center. Do you think that would work better for you?

<u>Mr. Washington</u>: Yes, sir. It surely would.

It was so simple! Why hadn't the other doctors figured it out?

The answer, I believe, is that the focus of doctors is on solving medical problems – in this case congestive heart failure – and we have gotten so good at it that getting to know about patients' lives is no longer considered essential. Now that diagnostic tests are so good and treatments so advanced, all that appears to be necessary is to order the right tests, make the correct diagnosis, recall or look up the appropriate treatment, and prescribe it. Getting to know patients as individuals is considered nice, if there is time, and even enjoyable sometimes, but not essential.

While supervising doctors in the clinic, I often suggested that they ask their patients to describe to them a typical day in their lives. But I could tell that most of them were thinking, *how is that going to help me decide which medicine to prescribe for their elevated blood pressure?*

A goal-directed approach requires an understanding of each person's life story and current situation. This information is absolutely essential because, unlike diseases, goals cannot be viewed in isolation from the person to whom they belong.

In the case of Mr. Washington, knowing that he had congestive heart failure and prescribing the correct medications was insufficient to improve his quality of life, which depended upon his ability to participate in morning activities with friends at the senior center. When I asked him what else he would like to be able to do, he said that he would love to be able to walk two blocks down to the drugstore where he used to visit friends on a regular basis. With that objective in mind, I was able to devise a strategy involving a relatively short-acting medicine, taken right before exertion, which made it possible for him to walk the two blocks without developing shortness of breath or chest pain. To my knowledge, he was able to stay out of the hospital for at least the next two years.

Maximization vs. Deficit Reduction

There is no theoretical limit to the amount of pleasure or meaning a person could derive from an activity, and it is always possible to improve performance – at least that is what I tell myself every time I play basketball. While helping people find the activities that would provide the most pleasure and meaning is probably beyond the scope of health care, helping people improve their performance could and probably should be.

Focusing directly on goal attainment would encourage the health care system to pay more attention to maximizing function rather than simply addressing functional deficits. This already occurs in rehabilitation settings, in sports medicine, and in mental health to some degree. Consider a saleswoman who wants to improve her already normal memory for names in order to perform beet on the job. Shouldn't she be able to come to a health care professional for advice and assistance?

The objective of problem-oriented health care is to bring everyone up to a minimum level of normal. A goal-oriented approach seeks to help people achieve the maximum possible quality of life. However, doing so does require helping people face the inevitable challenges that occur along the way.

Quality of Life and Unhealthy Behaviors

Many of the greatest challenges to better health in America involve unhealthy behaviors. Making the difficult choice to change a long-practiced behavior requires a very powerful reason. In my clinical experience, an essential first step is identifying a compelling quality of life goal. Sometimes, as in the case of Mrs. Gooch (Chapter 1), survival can provide sufficient motivation, but more often quality of life goals are more powerful.

Several years ago, my colleagues and I interviewed a number of people who had been able to lose at least 10% of their body weight and keep it off for more than a year. In every case, those people mentioned a specific quality of life goal that motivated them. Some wanted to be able to play tennis again or run marathons. Others wanted not to have to take medicines for diabetes or to have a joint replacement. And for others the motivation had to do with relationships, such as not being an embarrassment to their children or being able to play with their grandchildren.

Changing a lifelong behavior is really hard! It requires making a lifelong commitment, and it means giving up things that have given you pleasure. Your brain must break old neural connections and form new ones. You have to want something very badly to be willing to do make such a commitment and then go through the discomfort that will be involved in following through on it. The quality of life goal you choose must be compelling and long lasting. It has to be something important enough to carry you past temptation and prevent you from falling back into prior patterns of behavior.

The problem-oriented medical approach to overeating is to first label it – we now have specific categories: overweight, obese, and morbidly obese – and then to prescribe dietary modifications, physical activity, sometimes medications, and possibly even surgery to rectify to problem. The goal-directed approach would begin with a discussion of goals, followed by an assessment of resources (family support, access to healthy foods, ability to exercise, etc.) and then a thoughtful consideration of potential strategies.

Chronic Pain

Pain is a common impediment to quality of life, and the overuse and abuse of prescription pain medicines has become a major challenge for patients, doctors, and our society. When chronic pain is viewed as a problem, the solutions are directed at pain relief, and medical visits tend to focus on medication dosing and pain contracts.

A purely problem-oriented approach to chronic pain typically begins with determining the specific cause of the pain and the type of pain you are having – somatic, visceral, or neuropathic. Treatment is then determined based upon the cause and type of pain. It usually involves medicine but might also include physical therapy or complementary measures (e.g. massage, acupuncture, etc.).

I have found that conversations with patients with chronic pain are more productive when the focus is on goals. Typical questions I might ask are, "When we reduce the amount of pain you are having, how will your life be different?" "What do you hope to be able to do once you have less pain?" "What does the pain keep you from doing?"

Focusing on quality of life goals has at least two benefits. Setting quality of life goals can provide motivation for you to work harder on the things required for improvement (e.g. specific exercises, meditation, etc.). At the same time, pursuing a specific goal can focus your attention on something other than your pain. During visits with your doctor, discussing goals can change typically negative conversations into more positive, forward-looking ones.

Overdiagnosis

It might seem odd to suggest that making an accurate diagnosis is not always essential for deciding how to address a particular health challenge. Certainly many physicians would be concerned about this suggestion. However, I hope some of the examples I have provided have convinced you that a specific diagnosis is not always necessary. In fact, one clear benefit of a goal-directed approach to quality of life issues is reduction of unnecessary tests and treatments.

A number of years ago, while giving a talk at a national conference, my voice completely gave out. I couldn't make a sound for 15 or 20 minutes. When I got back home, I saw my primary care doctor, who referred me to an otorhinolaryngologist — an ear, nose, and throat doctor — who stuck a mirror deep into my throat and said that my vocal cords looked fine. He sent me on to a speech therapist who suggested a more sophisticated test, which involved videotaping the movement of my vocal cords.

Having just had my vocal cords examined, I wasn't thrilled about having it done again, so I asked the speech therapist what she thought might be wrong. I can no longer remember the name of the disorder she mentioned, but I do remember asking her how that condition would be treated. She said that if that was indeed the problem there was really nothing much that could be done, to which I replied, "Then I'd rather not know whether that's what I have." Her response was, "But we need a diagnosis." I respectfully disagreed, refused the procedure, and suggested to her that we assume it was not that condition and try some things that might be helpful. She reluctantly agreed, and my voice returned to normal with antihistamines for allergies, stress reduction techniques, and sips of water before and while lecturing.

I will bring up the subject of over-diagnosis again later in this book when I discuss the hazards of labeling. I also recommend that you consider reading the excellent book by Gilbert Welch called *Over-Diagnosed: Making People Sick in the Pursuit of Health.*

Overtreatment

Within a problem-oriented health care system, nearly everyone is incentivized to find and apply a treatment (solution), most often a medication. The biggest beneficiaries of this compulsion are the pharmaceutical companies.

Pharmaceutical companies wisely use goal-directed messages to promote their products. They know that most people are, by nature, goal-directed. For example, ads often show before-and-after sequences where people who had been sitting are later walking their dogs after taking the company's, say, arthritis medicine. Or they show an actress/patient with a relapsing neurological disorder now engaged in a wide variety of physical activities, as a velvety-voiced narrator says, "Imagine what you could do with fewer recurrences."

However, pharmaceutical companies also exploit the fact that we have been taught to think of our bodies as broken machines, even to the point of inventing new diagnoses with catchy acronyms to convince us that we need their new drugs. Recent examples include premenstrual dysphoric disorder (PMDD), overactive bladder syndrome (OBS), hypoactive sexual desire disorder (HSDD), menopausal sexual dysfunction (MSD), and opiate induced constipation (OIC).

What the pharmaceutical companies are banking on is that by giving common symptoms a diagnostic label, those symptoms become more significant, more treatment-worthy. In an ad for an expensive medicine used to treat dry eyes, for example, the actress/patient says that she was content to live with the symptoms until she learned that she had a *disease* called dry eyes syndrome!

Experts have estimated that three times as many children are receiving the diagnosis of attention deficit hyperactivity disorder than actually have the condition, and most of them are being treated for years with potentially hazardous amphetamine derivatives. Much of the fault for this lies with the pharmaceutical companies who have capitalized on the fears of parents that their children are at risk of falling behind their peers unless they take their medicines.

The typical pharmaceutical company sales pitch includes three messages: (1) your symptoms are caused by an actual *disease* that has a name; 2) you shouldn't have to tolerate them; and 3) there is a specific solution – just ask your doctor if you should take this powerful new medicine. This practice has been called "disease mongering," a term introduced by Lynn Payer in her book, *Disease-Mongers: How Doctors, Drug Companies, and Insurers are making You Feel Sick.* Ray Moynihan calls it "selling sickness" (In *Selling Sickness: How the World's Biggest Pharmaceutical Companies are Turning us all into Patients*).

Make no mistake: pharmaceutical companies are preying on your base fears. And this predatory behavior is reprehensible. As I write this book, the television advertisements for a particular class of new diabetes medicines illustrate the hazards of separating problem-solving from goal achievement.

We used to think that high blood sugar levels (diabetes) caused heart attacks and strokes. It now looks like inactivity, obesity, and genetics contribute to the development of inflammation in the blood vessels which leads to elevated blood pressure, cholesterol, and blood sugar levels. It is the inflammation and the elevations of blood pressure and cholesterol that then leads to heart attacks and strokes, not elevated blood sugar levels.

Put another way, we now believe that Type 2 diabetes and heart attacks/strokes have a common cause, rather than the former causing the latter. Therefore lowering blood sugar levels will not reduce your risk of a heart attack or stroke. Certain types of diabetes medicines do seem to reduce the risk of heart attacks, but it is probably due to other effects of those particular medicines and not to blood sugar reduction.

Elevated levels of sugar in the bloodstream can, over long periods of time, in susceptible individuals, cause blindness, kidney failure, nerve damage, and amputations. But these complications are uncommon and take many years to develop. For example, if you were to develop Type 2 diabetes at age 55, with an average blood sugar level of 212 (A1c of 9%), almost twice the normal level, and you did absolutely nothing at all to lower it, the chance that you would ever go blind or develop kidney failure would be less than 5%, and you would have a less than 10% chance of having an amputation.

However, if your average blood sugar level was 212, you probably wouldn't feel very good. When blood sugar levels rise above a certain level (usually around 200), sugar spills into the urine. The sugar molecules pull water and salt along with them, causing you to make too much urine. The result is that you become dehydrated, and that causes you to feel tired, weak, thirsty, and lightheaded. You may also have a dry mouth, dry eyes, dry skin, and constipation. These symptoms go away when blood sugar levels are reduced with diet, physical activity and medicines. In other words, lowering blood sugar levels can improve quality of life, but makes only a small contribution to prevention of premature death and disabilities.

All of this has been well-documented and should be well understood by the medical community. Nonetheless, as of the writing of this book, a newly developed class of diabetes medicines is being aggressively advertised on television. These medicines reduce blood sugar levels by increasing the amount of sugar passing into the urine. In other words, these drugs *contribute to* the process that causes the symptoms that bother people with diabetes!

Listen to the ads: "You may experience lightheadedness, fatigue, weakness, and dry mouth. And while it isn't a weight loss medicine, you might lose some weight." That's because *you will be dehydrated!*

Since symptom relief is a main reason for treating high blood sugar levels, these medicines are counterproductive. However, many doctors who prescribe these expensive new medicines are unaware that what they are doing makes no sense. After all, they are lowering blood sugar and A1c levels (i.e. managing the disease), which is what they were trained to do, and they are achieving the A1c target by which they are being judged and, increasingly, paid.

One ad concludes, "Imagine life with a lower A1c"—a strange imperative since the only ones likely to benefit, in this case, from *your* lower A1c are your doctor and the drug company.

This kind of harmful treatment can only occur in a system where a fixation on solving problems - a strategy – becomes disconnected from person-centered health objectives… quality of life… etc. – the goals

The Important Case of Coronary Artery Disease

A heart attack is an event in which the flow of blood, oxygen, and nutrients to a section of heart muscle is suddenly blocked by a blood clot. If flow is not restored quickly, that section of heart muscle can die or be permanently damaged. For years, the medical community assumed that the gradual narrowing of the coronary arteries – the blood vessels that nourish the heart muscle – led to reduced flow, then blood clotting, and heart attacks. Based on this assumption, cardiologists and cardiac surgeons developed techniques to either open up those narrowed arteries with balloons and stents, or to bypass the blockages with grafts.

We now know that our assumption about the cause of heart attacks was incorrect. It turns out that most heart attacks occur when a plaque on the inside wall of a coronary artery breaks open, leading to the formation of a clot that suddenly blocks the flow of blood through that artery. It turns out that clots are just as likely to occur in arteries with very little or no narrowing as in those that are narrowed to the point of reduced blood flow.

The gradual narrowing and blockage of coronary arteries can, however, cause pain with physical activity (angina). These new insights explains why opening up or bypassing partially blocked coronary arteries improves angina, but does very little to prevent heart attacks. There are a few situations in which opening up partially blocked coronary arteries prevents premature death (e.g., when all three vessels are blocked and the heart muscle has been weakened by prior heart attacks), but this may have nothing to do with prevention of heart attacks.

So, why are so many angioplasties and bypass surgeries still carried out on people with no symptoms?

The answer is of great concern not only to those who care about patient outcomes, but to those who pay for these expensive operations. In fact, some research has been done to try to figure it out, and there seem to be two reasons. Certainly physicians and hospitals have a large financial interest in performing these procedures. However, it is also clear that many cardiologists and cardiovascular surgeons simply don't believe the research findings and choose to ignore them. They still firmly believe that fixing the blood flow problem, restoring normal circulation to the heart muscle, ought to improve health. That is how they were trained to think, and it just makes sense – fix abnormalities and health will be restored.

The goal-directed approach to a patient with coronary artery disease would begin with a consideration of the impact, if any, of the condition on quality or length of life. For example, if an individual's quality of life was negatively impacted by chest pain during exertion, opening up the coronary arteries would be worth considering if other less invasive approaches (e.g. physical activity and medications) had not worked. If, on the other hand, the goal was to prolong life by preventing heart attacks, the more effective approach could include physical activity, a statin, low-dose aspirin, blood pressure control, and smoking cessation. In any case, the strategies would be clearly and explicitly related to patient goals and trade-offs would be acknowledged and discussed.

The Threshold Principle

As mentioned earlier, health challenges rarely have a single cause. We are all subject to thousands of risk factors. Some we were born with and some we have acquired since then. When enough risk factors are present, or when individual risk factors are significant enough, a *threshold* is reached or exceeded, and our health is challenged. This is sometimes called the *threshold principle*.

People who experience migraines know that a variety of factors can precipitate a headache, including stress, foods, medicines, change in barometric pressure, lack of sleep, bright lights, odors, hunger, and hormonal changes. However, they may not be aware that most of their headaches are the result of combinations of these factors, and that any one factor is not usually strong enough to have caused the headache by itself.

The truth is that given the combination of enough risk factors of sufficient strength, almost all of us would have a migraine headache. People who suffer migraines regularly either have a lower headache threshold, or they have more — or stronger — risk factors.

The threshold principle applies to nearly every health challenge you will face, from head colds to cancer. Even conditions that are the result of genetic mutations can be thought of in this way.

During my clinical career I took care of many people with sickle cell disease, a condition that is the result of a mutation in a single gene involved in making hemoglobin, the chemical in the blood that carries iron. Despite the fact that all of these patients had the same genetic mutation, some died in childhood, others were hospitalized repeatedly, still others avoided hospitalizations but were disabled, and many others grew up, completed their education, got married, and held regular steady jobs. How can these different outcomes be explained? The answer is that while they all had the same major risk factor - the genetic mutation, factors like income, education, family and social support, and other health challenges had an impact as well.

The best way I have found to address health challenges using the threshold principle is to make a list of the possible contributing factors and then identify the factors that can be reduced or eliminated. While it is not often possible to address all of the factors on the list, addressing some of them — even if they aren't the most significant ones — can reduce the combined impact of the risk factors below the *threshold* for the challenge we seek to address.

Some years ago I took care of an 80-year-old woman whose challenge was frequent falls. She lived alone in her own home, which she and her now-deceased husband had purchased 50 years earlier. Her goal was to continue to live independently in that house, even if it meant taking certain risks.

Together, she and I made a list of all the factors that might be contributing to her falls – medications, arthritis, environmental hazards, cataracts, calloused feet, worn out shoes, etc. I then helped her address the factors that we could address, including a referral for cataract surgery. The eye specialist called to say that, based upon the density of her cataracts, the surgery could be delayed a while longer. When I explained that the cataracts might be contributing to her falls, he agreed to remove them.

After the surgery, she was able to remain in her home until her death from other causes, and never, to my knowledge, suffered another serious fall.

Trade-Offs

Just as life prolonging measures often reduce quality of life, strategies to improve quality of life can sometimes shorten your life. For example, medicines that make you feel better but also affect your alertness or reaction speed (e.g., antihistamines, pain medications, muscle relaxants, etc.) can increase your risk of death from a car accident or fall. Antibiotics used to treat a self-limited infection like bronchitis or sinusitis can encourage the growth of antibiotic-resistant germs, which could cause a serious and difficult to treat infection in the future. A goal-directed approach doesn't resolve these conflicts, but it can help you to clarify the trade-offs you are making.

Mr. Menninger was an 88-year-old retired minister who had developed Alzheimer's disease. He also had high blood pressure, high cholesterol, a heart valve abnormality, and a heart rhythm disturbance (atrial fibrillation). He was referred to me by his cardiologist, who had provided excellent problem-oriented medical care. When I met Mr. Menninger, his cholesterol level was normal; his heart rate was well-controlled; he was on all of the right anticoagulant and blood pressure medications; but his quality of life was terrible, and it was getting progressively worse. In addition to memory loss, he was lightheaded to the point of falling, and he was too drowsy to sit in church without falling asleep. His wife was afraid to take him for a walk for fear he would fall and she wouldn't be able to get him back up. He was no longer able to make even simple decisions.

Mr. Menninger's wife was certain that he would not want his life to be extended, particularly since his dementia was going to gradually get worse. We therefore focused our efforts on improving his quality of life. Stopping his blood pressure medicines reduced his lightheadedness and improved his ability to stay awake. There were no more falls. He rejoined his Sunday school class and was able, on several occasions, to give the closing prayer. Mr. Menninger lived another year in relative peace and happiness, before dying of complications of his heart disease. There is no way to know whether he would have lived longer if he had continued to take the blood pressure medicines.

Trade-offs can also be important when thinking about short-term versus long-term quality of life. For example, if you have an episode of back pain, "killing" the pain completely might allow you to do things that could cause further injury or delay healing, resulting in further damage and greater back trouble down the road. The problem-oriented approach views pain as something to be eradicated when possible. In the goal-directed approach, however, pain is viewed within the context of your health goals, that is, what you are trying to achieve in both the short- and long-term.

Prevention and Quality of Life

In addition to the standard list of preventive measures discussed in Chapter 1, there are things that you can do now to assure that you will be able to do the things you enjoy in the future.

For example, if the things you enjoy doing depend upon being able to think clearly, you should consider brain-preserving behaviors like physical activity, reading and studying, and social activities, and you should consider trying to reduce your risk of brain damage from a head injury (e.g., use your seat belts and bicycle helmet), a stroke (e.g., consider blood pressure reduction and low-dose aspirin), and excessive consumption of alcohol.

If your favorite activities require good vision, you might consider wearing protective goggles when doing tasks that could result in eye injury, wearing ultraviolet protective glasses when spending time in the sunshine, and having periodic eye check-ups to be sure you aren't developing glaucoma.

We now know that the hearing loss that affects many older people is caused or accelerated by repeated exposure to loud noises. So, if your hearing is important to you, you should try to avoid exposure to loud noises and wear hearing protection when noise exposure is unavoidable.

In summary, maintaining, improving, and preserving health-related quality of life are goals for nearly everyone, but each person's definition of quality of life is different. Simply eradicating problems won't necessarily improve quality of life. A goal-directed approach can often be more effective because it focuses directly on the outcomes that matter and encourages consideration of a wider variety of potential strategies. It can also help clarify the inevitable trade-offs you will make between quality and quantity of life.

**WHAT GOAL-DIRECTED CARE
WOULD LOOK LIKE – PART 2**

1. The health risk survey you would complete each year (See Part 1) would also collect information about what you enjoyed doing and what you would like to be able to do but can't. Then, at your annual visit with your primary care team, you would discuss potential strategies for maintaining and enhancing your quality of life.

2. As new health challenges occurred, you would discuss them with your primary health care team, always focusing on how they are affecting your ability to participate in essential and meaningful life activities.

3. Your progress would be measured by determining how well you were able to engage in the activities that make life worthwhile for you.

CHAPTER 3:

Personal Growth and Development

"Live as if you were to die tomorrow. Learn as if you were to live forever."

—*Mahatma Gandhi*

"Our only purpose in life is growth."

—*Elizabeth Kubler-Ross*

I often asked medical students and residents-in-training, "Aside from differences in the subject matter, how is being a doctor different from being an auto mechanic?"

They almost never come up with a valid answer — in fact, they are often speechless, and look at me like I'm crazy. But I'm persistent. I give them the most obvious hint: "How are people different from cars?"

This generates several predictable responses, such as "People have emotions," "People don't always cooperate," and, most disturbingly, "People can sue you."

Rarely have I encountered a doctor in training who is able to articulate that, unlike cars, people have goals. We are able to grow and develop physically, psychologically, and spiritually in response to the interactions we have with others and our environment. In fact, for humans, good health always involves the experience of personal growth and development.

To be fair, some auto mechanics develop relationships of a sort with some cars and with their drivers, and some mechanics are goal-directed. In fact, some cars - think race car, for example – grow and develop over time, but they are passive recipients of the actions taken by the mechanic. They are not actively involved and don't experience the changes. The goals and strategies are determined by the owner and mechanic, not the car.

While we normally think of growth and development as primarily a childhood concern, it is actually a lifelong process with at least two major components: (1) achievement of major developmental tasks, and (2) the ongoing process of becoming more resilient, adaptable, and capable of handling challenges. A goal-directed health care system would take both these components of into consideration for every patient, at every age.

Developmental Tasks

The table below contains a list of the major developmental tasks and the ages at which they tend to be accomplished, as proposed by the renowned developmental psychologists Erik and Joan Erikson.

DEVELOPMENTAL TASK	RELEVANT QUESTION	AGES WHEN FACED
Trust (vs. mistrust)	Can I trust the world and especially the people in it?	Birth – 2 years
Autonomy (vs. shame and doubt)	Is it OK to be me?	2 – 4 years
Initiative (vs. guilt)	Is it OK for me to do, move, and act?	4 – 5 years
Competence (vs. inferiority/ inadequacy)	Can I make it in the world?	5 – 12 years
Identity (vs. role confusion/ uncertainty)	Who am I? Who can I become?	13 – 19 years
Intimacy (vs. isolation)	Can I love?	20 – 24 years or 20 – 39 years
Generativity (vs. stagnation)	Can I make my life count?	25 – 64 years or 40 – 64 years
Ego integrity (vs. despair)	Is it OK to have been me?	65 years – death

Each developmental task builds upon the prior ones, which means that the earliest tasks are the most critical ones. Individuals who don't develop a sense of trust during their first three years of life will likely have difficulty forming relationships and dealing with losses throughout their lives. It is therefore appropriate that pediatric care focuses heavily on this goal, and that social programs have been developed to insure that we all experience optimal growth and development during early childhood. This is an area in which the current health care system is already, to some degree, goal-directed though more could certainly be done.

Unfortunately, developmental tasks receive much less attention in adults. In fact, adult developmental challenges are more often viewed as mental health problems — such as anxiety, depression, mid-life crisis, etc. But if optimal development throughout life was viewed as a goal, clinicians would be more likely to take a positive, proactive approach, and developmental challenges would be considered within the context of each person's entire life—past, present, and future—rather than as isolated events.

I am reminded of a 40-year-old woman and her 70-year-old mother, both patients of mine, the mother for more than 25 years. Since the death of her father while a teenager, the daughter had lived with her mother. Whenever she tried to become more independent — get a job, go on dates, etc. — the mother's many physical symptoms – headaches, dizziness, stomach pain, fatigue - became worse.

Once I began taking care of the daughter, the situation

became clearer to me. At each visit, I spent time teaching them how to contribute to the other's psychological growth. By focusing on personal development as a goal, I was able to help the daughter find the courage to get a job, move out, and get married (the identity and intimacy tasks) and the mother to proudly let her (the generativity and ego identity tasks).

Becoming More Resilient, Adaptable, and Capable of Handling Challenges
Physical Resilience

The most obvious example of physical resilience involves the immune system, the system in our bodies that recognizes and eliminates harmful germs, toxins, and cancer cells. Without doing anything at all, your immune system becomes more effective as you grow into adulthood. Each encounter with potentially harmful things in your environment naturally prepares you for subsequent encounters, assuming you don't die from the first encounter. ("What doesn't kill you makes you stronger.")

There are three ways to support the development of a strong immune system. First, help it thrive by practicing healthy behaviors. Eat a healthy diet, stay physically active, get sufficient sleep, manage stress, avoid tobacco products, and don't drink alcohol to excess.

Second, allow most exposures to happen. We suspect that children raised in the cleanest households are more likely to develop allergies including asthma, and we have very good evidence that early exposure to peanuts prevents later development of peanut allergies. So, resist the temptation to sterilize every surface in your house in an attempt to prevent infections. Instead wash your hands when you think you have been exposed to an infection like colds and the flu.

Finally, when minor infections occur, give your immune system a chance to respond before taking an antibiotic. Most viral infections of the eyes, nose, and throat get better just as quickly with or without antibiotics. So do bacterial infections like ear infections, sinus infections and bronchitis. Unless you have a condition that puts you at higher risk from these infections, it is generally safe to wait at least 5 – 7 days to see if your body can handle them itself, becoming more resilient in the process.

And don't forget that immunizations are a great way to promote physical resilience. Exposure to fragments of germs or germs that have been modified to reduce their ability to cause harm allows your immune system to develop resistance to infections that could actually kill you or make you very sick.

Psychological Resilience

Drs. Edward Deci and Richard Ryan have proposed that optimal growth and development are most likely to occur when three basic psychological needs are met, the need to feel connected to others (relationship), the need to believe we can accomplish achieve goals we set for ourselves (competence), and the need to feel that we can make personal decisions that matter (autonomy).

The implications of these principles are explained in laymen's language in a book by Daniel Pink called *Drive: The Surprising Truth about what Motivates Us.*

A goal-directed approach to health care would support all three psychological needs. Goal setting and strategic planning foster a more equal and collaborative relationship between doctors and patients. The assumption is that you are able to set and achieve goals, building your sense of competence, and you would clearly be in charge of any decisions that were made, supporting the need to feel autonomous.

Because the elimination of physical abnormalities becomes more and more difficult as we age, the problem-oriented paradigm encourages us to view aging negatively. However, as we have seen, growth and development continues to be a goal throughout life and may actually be enhanced by the experience of losses. In fact, some have argued that it is impossible to experience optimal growth and development without such experiences.

A goal-directed approach encourages us to think more positively about aging. If, as the World Health Organization believes, health is a state of well-being, and not the absence of problems, then there is no reason why older people can't be just as healthy as or healthier than younger people.

Functional Resilience

Since growth requires learning, it should not be surprising that experts in adult education have identified some of the components of adaptability and resilience, which, as it turns out, apply equally well to health and health care. Reframed for health they include: 1) the knowledge and skills required for healthy living; 2) the motivation to maintain and improve health; 3) integration within a social network and the relational skills necessary to do that; and 4) the habits of self-assessment, reflection, goal-setting, and self-directed learning.

Goal-directedness encourages greater personal responsibility. When we commit to a set of goals, we are more motivated to learn about how our bodies work and how to get the help we need than when we allow medical professionals to set the agenda for us.

Consider the following example. Doctors often have trouble deciding what to do for patients with common colds, bronchitis, and sinus infections. They feel pressure to prescribe antibiotics, even though they know that, aside from their placebo effect, antibiotics don't really help. Visits for these conditions often include a lecture about viruses and antibiotics and implied criticism for coming in for a self-limited condition.

As I began to adopt a goal-directed approach, I learned to take a different approach. I first tried to determine why the person came to see me, and what they hoped to achieve as a result of the visit – their short-term quality of life objectives. After trying to address those needs, I made sure they knew how to avoid spreading the infection to others and how to keep from getting similar infections in the future. When there was time, I asked about stress, sleep, and diet, factors that can affect resistance to infections. All of this typically took no more than 10 minutes but resulted, I hope, in a more knowledgeable patient who was motivated to improve their health habits – the growth and development goal.

As I became fully goal-directed, I began to view each patient encounter as an educational, motivational, and relation-ship-strengthening event for both patient and doctor instead of a one-time illness event requiring a solution.

The groundbreaking psychologist, Carl Rogers (1902-1987) found that all counseling strategies were effective to the extent that the counselor demonstrated all of the following: 1) genuineness (openness and self-disclosure); 2) acceptance (unconditional positive regard), and 3) empathy (ability to listen and express an understanding of the person's experi-ence). He subsequently concluded that those same behaviors were necessary for optimal interactions between all human beings. Robert Carcuff subsequently proposed that, in addi-tion to the three Rogerian principles, helping another person requires helping them to set goals and devise strategies to achieve them. Because we are social beings and because we thrive when helping others, optimal human growth and development requires mastery of those same skills.

In summary, a goal-directed approach to health and health care would support optimal growth and development, both directly by acknowledging specific developmental goals and objectives, and indirectly by reshaping interactions between patients and health care professionals. Health challenges would always be considered within the context of each patient's life trajectory, and including optimal growth and development as a goal would make it possible to view aging in a more positive light.

WHAT GOAL-DIRECTED CARE
WOULD LOOK LIKE – PART 3

1. Your primary care doctor would evaluate your growth and development from birth until death by asking you additional questions, and by observing your behavior every time you visited his or her office.

2. Decisions regarding medical interventions would be considered within the context of physical growth and development. For example, antibiotics might be delayed when safe to do so to allow the immune system to learn to deal with the offending germ.

3. Using counseling techniques and educational strategies, your doctor would help you achieve your developmental milestones and become more knowledgeable, adaptable, and resilient – able to handle the health challenges sure to come.

4. The care provided to you would be grounded in your relationship with your primary care doctor and designed to help you to become more competent to make good health care decisions and to achieve your health goals.

CHAPTER 4:
A Good Death

"Death is a process to be lived not a problem to be solved. Yet literally every clinician my wife and I have interacted with is more afraid of death than we are; they focus on solving the problems of our illness with little awareness of how we want to live our lives."

—Stuart Farber, MD, a family doctor in Seattle, Washington shortly before his death

The enemy is not death. The enemy is inhumanity. (paraphrased)

—D.G. Benfield, a pediatrician in Akron, Ohio

Dying Well

Discussions about death and dying rarely occur during routine doctor visits. When they do occur, it is usually in the context of a life-threatening illness, typically in the hospital, long after every treatment approach has failed and death is imminent.

This is because, in the current medical paradigm, death is the enemy. When a person dies, it represents a failure of medical care. Death represents defeat. That perspective makes it difficult for physicians, patients, and families to have frank and open conversations about how and where they would like to die. It also leads to unwarranted and unwanted aggressive measures to keep people alive, often to the bitter end.

Some physicians argue that they would spend more time discussing death and dying if they could be paid for the time required. However, several months after Medicare authorized payment for conversations about end-of-life preferences, a poll of 736 physicians conducted by three large non-profit organizations found that only 14% of them had ever billed for this service.

Since we all will die at some point, it makes sense for us to do what we can to insure that the circumstances surrounding our deaths will conform to our personal beliefs and preferences. One of the goals of health and health care should therefore be to increase the probability of a good death. If a good death was acknowledged to be a universal goal, it would no longer be a taboo subject. In fact, conversations regarding end-of-life preferences would begin early in adulthood and continue through the dying process.

The National Academy of Medicine has defined a good death as "one that is free from avoidable distress and suffering, for patients, family, and caregivers; in general accord with the patients' and families' wishes; and reasonably consistent with clinical, cultural, and ethical standards." And the well-known medical ethicists E. J. and L. L. Emanuel have proposed six categories of modifiable factors that may contribute to the quality of the dying process: 1) physical symptoms, 2) psychological and other mental factors, 3) economic and caregiving needs, 4) social relationships and support, 5) spiritual beliefs, and 6) hopes and expectations. The relative importance of these factors varies a great deal from person to person and situation to situation.

Advance Directives

Some end of life preferences can be expressed on standard legal forms. While the rules vary somewhat from state to state, all states now provide the opportunity for citizens to complete some sort of advance directive for health care. These documents are sometimes called "living wills." Since you don't know when death will come, *every adult* should strongly consider completing one of these documents.

While advance directives are often associated with old age, they are actually more important for younger adults whose deaths are more likely to create controversy. Perhaps the most notable examples have involved Karen Ann Quinlan and Terri Schiavo.

Karen Ann Quinlan was 21 years old in 1975 when she took a combination of a pain killer, an anti-anxiety drug, and alcohol, and lapsed into a persistent coma. Despite her parents' request, doctors refused to take her off of the respirator. The resulting legal battle resulted in new regulations requiring ethics committees in all hospitals, among other things.

Terri Schiavo was 26 when she had a cardiac arrest at her home in Florida, possibly caused by a low potassium level resulting from bulimia. Although she was successfully resuscitated by paramedics, she suffered severe brain damage and became totally dependent, requiring a feeding tube for nutrition. Schiavo's husband and legal guardian believed that she would not want be kept alive in that condition and requested that her feeding tube be removed, but her parents argued that she always had a strong will to live and would want life support continued. While the legal battle raged, health care professionals attempted speech and physical therapy and other experimental therapies, hoping to return her to a state of awareness, without success. Finally, after 15 years of bitter legal and eventually political strife, the feeding tube was removed and she was allowed to die.

Neither Karen Ann Quinlan nor Terri Schiavo had completed an advance directive. Had they done so, it would have made life much easier for their families and, to the degree they were aware of their own discomfort, for them.

Most formal advance directive documents allow you to document whether you would want to be resuscitated if you had a terminal illness and were expected to die with or without resuscitation within 6 months or were in a persistent coma. Many advance directives also ask about whether you would want to be fed through a tube or intravenous catheter. That becomes especially important in several U.S. states, which have decided that providing food and fluids is part of basic care and required unless there is a specific directive to do otherwise.

Advance directives also make it possible to designate a surrogate decision-maker in case you are unable to make decisions for yourself. In many, if not most cases this may be the most important part of the document but only if that person knows your goals and preferences.

All states also allow you to create a *durable* power of attorney (DPOA) for health care, in which you can specify who you want to make health care decisions for you if you are unable to speak for yourself. Unlike a regular power of attorney, a DPOA remains in effect after you have been declared incompetent to make decisions for yourself. Reminders, educational materials, assistance, and documentation of these legal expressions of your values and preferences ought to be provided and promoted in all primary care practices.

Currently, by federal law, health care providers who accept Medicare or Medicaid must inform you that you have a right to accept or refuse medical or surgical treatment and the right to execute an "advance directive." They must then ask you whether or not you have an advance directive. If the answer is "no," however, there is no requirement to ask if you would like help completing one. And if the answer is "yes," there is no requirement that you be asked to provide them with a copy of your directive to be put into your medical record.

Using electronic health records data, colleagues of mine recently estimated that the percentage of primary care medical records containing an advance directive was less than 5%. And a word of caution: Even if you have an advance directive in your outpatient medical records, that by no means guarantees that your directive will be available to the doctors who care for you in the hospital. Make sure you have a copy posted on your refrigerator for the emergency medical team and that your family members and caregivers have copies as well.

A goal-directed approach would assure that every competent person would be encouraged to complete all of the advance directive documents available in their state as early in their adult life as possible. Copies would be kept in all accessible medical records and by all family decision-makers.

Informal Directives

As important as they are, formal advance directive documents are not as important as the informal discussions you should have with close family members and your primary care physician. In my experience, the decisions that have to be made near the end of life rarely fall into the simple categories covered by advance directive forms. If you are still able to make your own decisions right up until your death, things are more likely to go the way you want them to. But if you are not, responsibility will fall to surrogate decision-makers – family, close friends, doctors, or ethics committees. If your goal is to have a "good death" as you define it, you need to make sure those people know your values and preferences.

Suggestions about how to initiate those conversations can be found at *http://www.dyingmatters.org/page/resources-talking-about-death-and-dying* and in the "Five Wishes" section of the "Aging with Dignity" website (*www.agingwithdignity*.org).

There is also a wonderful game families or friends can play called "My Gift of Grace" *(www.mygiftofgrace.com)*, developed at the Pennsylvania State Hershey Medical Center, which can help both you and your potential surrogate decision-makers discover your (and their) values and preferences about end-of-life care.

A variety of non-legal documents have also been created to help you think about your values and preferences more generally. One example is the Values History developed at the University of New Mexico: (*http://c.ymcdn.com/sites/www. hospicefed.org/resource/resmgr/hpcfm_pdf_doc/valueshistoryform. pdf*).

A goal-directed approach to health and health care would require you to think about your values, which, together with your resources, challenges, and preferences, are the basis for your health goals. Yes, goal-directed care would require more from you than problem-oriented care. It is, after all, your life and health we are talking about.

Values Pertaining to End-of-Life Care

In Chapter 1 I mentioned that my partners and I asked a number of questions of every new patient who enrolled in our geriatric practice over a period of 10 years. In addition to the questions discussed in that chapter, we also asked patients to choose, from a list of 14, the three values pertaining to end-of-life care they considered most important. The items came from a "Values History" developed by D. J. Doukas and L. B. McCullough. The results are shown in this table.

VALUE STATEMENT	% OF PEOPLE INCLUDING IT IN THEIR TOP 3
Thinking clearly	64%
Not being a burden to family	45%
Avoiding unnecessary pain and suffering	37%
Maintaining good relationships with family	28%
Maintain dignity until death	28%
Making own decisions	23%
Being treated with respect	17%
Feeling safe and secure	16%
Leaving good memories	15%
Being comfortable when dying	9%
Being with loved ones at death	7%
Having religious beliefs respected	7%
Contributing to medical research	4%
Having my body respected after death	0%

What are your top three end-of-life values? Could your potential surrogate decision-makers guess which ones you chose? Can you see how it might be helpful if they could?

Trade-Offs

Just as there are often trade-offs between length and quality of life goals, there are trade-offs to be considered between staying alive and having a good death.

When asked how they would prefer to die, most people say "in my sleep." Death during sleep is most likely to result from a heart attack or stroke. Therefore measures to reduce the risk of heart attacks and strokes reduce the likelihood of that kind of "peaceful" death. There might, therefore, come a point in your life when you should decide to stop treating your high blood pressure and cholesterol. There is no simple solution to this dilemma, but it is worth thinking about with your physician, particularly when your life expectancy is limited.

Even more challenging choices must often be made when faced with a life threatening condition like cancer. Atul Gawande, in his book *Being Mortal*, does a wonderful job of explaining and suggesting ways to address these choices. For example, he suggests that people who are dying should consider four questions: 1) What is your understanding of the situation and its potential outcomes? 2) What are your fears and hopes? 3) What trade-offs are willing and unwilling to make? and 4) What course of action best serves this understanding?

The balance between relief of pain and preserving the ability to think is often an issue at the end of life. In most cases, it is an issue that can be discussed when the time comes. But it can be helpful to have thought about it ahead of time and to have discussed your thoughts with your doctor and family members.

On this subject of trade-offs involved in planning for a good death, a particularly interesting case, about which I was informally consulted, involved a couple who had been married for 50 years. The husband tended to avoid doctors until he was seriously ill. Clinic visits almost always resulted in hospitalizations. He had survived a series of heart attacks and strokes but was still able to function as the local director of the American Association of Retired People (AARP).

His wife, on the other hand, saw her family physician nearly every other week. Her symptoms varied from visit to visit and always seemed to resolve with time and reassurance. However, when she saw blood in her urine, and a urine test confirmed it, she was advised to have additional tests to determine the cause.

When she asked her doctor what the tests might reveal, he mentioned the possibility of cancer. At that point she stated emphatically that she didn't want the tests. When asked why, she began to cry, saying, "I've been so afraid that my husband would die and leave me all alone. You know he has almost died several times already. My greatest hope is that I will die first. If I have cancer, that would be a blessing! Let's hope that is what it is."

That, of course, led to a long-overdue discussion with her physician (which might have prevented many of her previous symptoms and medical visits). He encouraged her to talk with her husband. She finally did agree to further testing, which showed that the bleeding was not due to cancer.

What Goal-Directed Care
Would Look Like – Part IV

1. At annual visits with your primary health care team, your advance directives, both formal (Living Will, Durable Power of Attorney, Do not Resuscitate Document) and informal (expressed values and preferences), would be reviewed and updated.

2. Your primary care doctors would provide you with a checklist of things to do to prepare for a good death. This would include, for example, discussing with family members your values and preferences regarding end of life care, how you feel about autopsy and organ donation, making sure someone knows where you keep your important documents, and selecting a funeral home and burial plot or crematorium.

3. Your progress toward goal achievement would be measured by completion of the advance directives and preparatory tasks.

4. As you aged, you and your physician would speak frequently about death, not as a problem to be avoided at all costs, but as a fundamental part of life.

SECTION 2:
Obstacles and Challenges

"All our knowledge has its origins in our perceptions."

—Leonardo da Vinci

"You can't change the fruit without changing the root."

—Stephen R. Covey

I'm hoping that, at this point in the book, you are thinking, "This is so obvious. Why does he even need to write a book about it?" Hang on. I'm about to tell you.

When I explain goal-directed care to doctors, their first response is usually, "We already do that." Once I have convinced them that they don't, they say, "It isn't possible."

By the way, it isn't hard to convince them that they aren't practicing some aspects of goal-directed care. All I have to do is show them their low rates of delivery of high impact primary and secondary preventive services, the lack of recorded information about their patients' daily activities, and the low rates of documentation of patients' advance directives.

It would be difficult, but not impossible, for physicians to implement goal-directed care. They would need additional training, a different record keeping system, more advanced decision-support tools, and a different billing process. Delivering goal-directed care would also require a different kind of primary care team and better information about how to help people achieve their goals. Gathering that type of information would probably require new research methods.

However, I know that it is possible for health care professionals to use many of the principles of goal-directed care. As much as anything, it is a mindset, a different way of thinking. Once you have adopted that mindset, it is possible to provide goal-directed care even within a problem-oriented system.

More to the point of this book, it is very possible for you to obtain goal-directed health care from our problem-oriented health care system, but, to do so, you will need to understand some things about how health care professionals think and the constraints within which they must practice. My experience suggests that the information I have provided in this section will be important to you. I have made it as brief and interesting as I could. However, I won't be offended if you decide it is too technical, and you skip to Section 3.

CHAPTER 5:

Different Ways of Looking at Things

"The world as we have created it is a process of our thinking. It cannot be changed without changing our thinking."

—*Albert Einstein*

Paradigms

Goal-directed health care could be considered to be a paradigm shift. The word "paradigm" refers to the set of assumptions, concepts, and perspectives that determine how we make sense of what we observe. For example, some people think of our country as a huge corporation, while others see it as an extended family. Those different perspectives have implications for what kinds of leaders we vote for and what sorts of laws we support.

As time passes, science advances, and circumstances change, paradigms come in and go out of favor. Physicist Thomas Kuhn pointed out that we tend to cling tightly to paradigms for as long as possible even when it is obvious they are no longer consistent with our observations or needs. For example, we still teach standard Newtonian physics in high school before introducing relativity even though we know that relativity is a more accurate way to understand how the world works. Why not teach the most accurate model first and then explain that Newtonian physics is a useful approximation?

Because so much has been invested in an existing paradigm, those with influence and those who are benefitting most from it try to shore it up as long as they can with a series of tweaks – smallish corrections, which provide reassurance that major changes won't be necessary. Eventually the tweaks result in absurdities obvious to those outside the system even when those within the system can't yet see them.

There are many examples of this in the criminal justice system. Consider the following. Individuals caught *in the act* of committing serious crimes can be released based upon errors made by police officers during the arrest or investigation. Individuals willing to admit that they participated in a criminal act are *required* to commit perjury by pleading innocent in order to be allowed to have a trial. Although many crimes are complex (e.g., cybercrimes, financial crimes, medical malpractice, etc.), the process used to select juries, by design, tends to result in panels of people with little or no expertise in the subject matter. And, while the system trusts jurors to make critical decisions about guilt and innocence, sometimes life or death, jurors are not allowed to hear many categories of potentially relevant information (e.g. information about previous crimes) for fear it might bias their decisions.

While to those of us outside of the criminal justice system these practices seem odd and even absurd, those within the system (e.g. attorneys and judges) defend them, providing all of the reasons why they make perfect sense.

The major tenets of modern medicine were developed during the mid-1800s. This was a time when classification systems for plants and animals were being developed based upon a new understanding of genetics and natural selection. Autopsies became legal, and signs and symptoms could be correlated directly with the abnormalities that caused them. It is not surprising then that the paradigm directing health care was built upon the following assumptions:

Health is characterized by the absence of abnormalities. To achieve health, we must then correct, eliminate, and/or control these abnormalities.

Health care professionals, because of their extensive training in the medical sciences, are the legitimate experts in the detection and correction of abnormalities.

It is the responsibility of patients to be alert to symptoms and signs that things are not normal, report them to a health care professional, listen to the advice provided, and follow it.

Note: The relatively recent shift from paternalism – doctors telling patients what to do – to the now-popular concept of shared decision-making, in which all options are presented to patients who then make the final decisions about how to proceed, is an example of a paradigm tweak. It doesn't change the underlying paradigm. It just makes doctors and patients feel better about it.

So, what's wrong with this way of looking at health and health care? After all, it has resulted in tremendous advances in medical science, which have contributed to increases in life expectancy and quality of life.

Shortcomings of the Current Paradigm

For one thing, the spectrum of health challenges has changed dramatically since the mid-1800s. Because of immunizations, antibiotics, and the aging of the population, many more health care dollars are now spent on management of chronic (long-term) conditions like coronary artery disease, chronic kidney disease, arthritis, and dementia than on acute (short-term) illnesses and injuries like infections and broken bones.

We have also become so good at identifying and correcting abnormalities that we need to determine which abnormalities are important, and which can be followed or ignored. The concept of prioritization has gained importance. Expectations have also been raised. People used to wait until they were near death to consult a doctor; now the focus is on prevention and early detection, concepts that were never part of the original paradigm.

We have also begun to realize that, despite the successes of the problem-solving approach, we seem to have somehow lost the human aspects of health care embedded in traditional doctor-patient relationships. The system often seems better designed to meet the needs of health care professionals and health care institutions than the needs of those they are supposed to be helping.

Labeling

Problem-oriented thinking encourages the categorization of health-related differences as either normal or abnormal. People with higher than average blood pressures are *hypertensive*, those with higher than average blood sugar levels are *diabetic*. Such labels are helpful to physicians, since they help direct treatment decisions, but they can be harmful to patients.

In a classic Canadian study, workers randomly assigned to a group that was screened and informed about their elevated blood pressures were more likely to miss work over the next 6 months than those in the group that was screened but not told the results. To make matters worse, the blood pressures of those who were told were not any lower after 6 months than the blood pressures of those who were not told. Five years later, the average salaries of workers who were told they had high blood pressure (again, completely randomly) were lower than the salaries of those who were not told. Simply being labeled hypertensive ended up leading to negative health and financial outcomes for some of the individuals involved.

In another small study, a medical student and I found that people who had been given the diagnosis of high blood pressure believed that it took them twice as long to recover from a cold compared to other adults of the same age and gender.

Since blood pressure and viral infections should in no way be related, the most likely explanation is that those given the diagnosis of high blood pressure considered themselves to be less healthy generally.

Approximately one-third of premature deaths are now the result of unhealthy behaviors including cigarette smoking, abuse of alcohol and drugs, lack of exercise, and poor eating habits. Viewing these behaviors as "problems" has unfortunately not been very effective for helping people change them. And, as with the labeling of risk factors, labeling can be harmful.

For example, we still have a very limited understanding of what causes some people to weigh more than other people. And while being heavier is associated with certain medical conditions like diabetes, that association only applies to some people. Being called overweight or obese is more likely to make people feel worse about themselves than it is to result in sustained weight loss.

Care of the Elderly: The Canary in the Mine

Primarily because of advances in public health rather than medicine, life expectancy in the U.S. has increased by 30 years in the past century. As we age, the adverse physical consequences of injuries, illnesses, and the aging process accumulate. As a result, aging, for most Americans, is associated with more doctor visits, more tests and procedures, and more medicines. Most people over 85 visit a doctor at least 15 times per year, and most people over 65 take more than 6 different medications regularly.

Because doctors keep getting better at identifying abnormalities, the cost of care continues to increase at an unsustainable rate, particularly for the elderly. As a stopgap measure, policy makers have reduced the amounts they are willing to pay health care professionals, who already don't want to see older patients because of their complexity. Those of us who have focused our careers on the care of older adults are appalled by the generally poor quality of care that the elderly receive.

The failure of the health care system to meet the needs of the elderly should be viewed as a warning signal, like the canary in the coal mine whose death from carbon monoxide and methane gas exposure was a warning to the miners to get out of the mine. It should alarm all of us sufficiently that we act to overhaul our health care system before it becomes any more toxic and dysfunctional than it already is.

There have been other warning signals, to which the health care system has generally responded with tweaks. Decades ago, women said they didn't want pregnancy to be treated like a problem. Through their efforts, birth settings and prenatal education have improved, though problem-oriented obstetrical care is still the underlying paradigm. The hospice and palliative care movement resulted from the inability of the health care system to adequately address the needs of those in the process of dying. It resulted in an almost separate branch of health care for people at the end of life, with its own set of health care professionals, its own admission criteria, and its own payment structure. I'll say a bit more about this in the next chapter.

Where Does the Problem-Oriented Approach Lead?

As more and more is known about the human genome, and as genomic testing becomes more affordable, there will soon be pressure for everyone to have their DNA mapped early in life. The term, "personalized medicine," is being used to describe the brave new world of precision therapy based upon one's genetic makeup.

It is also possible to modify genes by inserting or removing small pieces of DNA. This technique, called CRISPR, is already being used experimentally to cure a few inherited diseases like cystic fibrosis. Once that is possible, it will also be theoretically possible to change other genetic traits. For example, it might be possible to increase adult height or reduce the risk of being overweight as an adult by genetically modifying a fetus or young child. At that point, who will we allow to decide which traits are normal and abnormal?

A problem-oriented view of health and health care depends upon the elimination of abnormalities, and the better we get at doing that, the more we tighten our definitions of normal. Diabetes used to be defined as a fasting blood sugar above 140; now it only has to be above 126.

The long term survival of human beings depends upon genetic diversity. The quest for normality leads us in the direction of a perfect genome. However, the closer we come to that objective, the greater the risk of human extinction due to a resistant infection or change in our environment. Sickle cell disease exists because the sickle cell gene protected those affected from the malaria parasite. The strategies employed in problem-oriented health care only make sense if they aren't very successful. The quest for normalcy only makes sense if we can't accomplish it.

Some of you might want to argue that goal-directedness could lead us to the same place. Doesn't everyone want to live forever, play quarterback for the Patriots, run a billion dollar company, write the next great American novel, and star in a successful rock band? Actually, no; they don't. In fact, a goal-directed approach would result in greater diversity since the unique skills of each individual would be celebrated, and survival, as I have said, isn't just an individual concept. If we are ever able to completely eliminate death, both individual and societal goal-setting would take on even greater importance. Some have speculated that, in such a situation, dying rather than surviving would then become the predominant goal.

Change is Hard

While goal-directed health care requires only a small, logical change in perspective, it has been interesting for me to watch how hard it is for health care professionals to understand it. Common mistakes and misconceptions include:

1. Beginning with a problem; then asking about goals. ("The goal for your diabetes should be to ..." or "The goal will be to get your pain under control..." rather than "If we can get your blood sugar down, you may

feel well enough to play basketball... or when your pain is under better control, perhaps you can return to work.")

2. Confusing goals with strategies and objectives (controlling blood pressure is a strategy; preventing strokes is an objective; the goal is prevent premature death and disability)

3. Focusing only on quality of life goals, neglecting survival, personal growth and development, and preparation for a good death;

4. Assuming the patient is entirely responsible for articulating goals, when, in fact, goal-setting and developing a plan for achievement should be collaborative;

The good news is that, while goal-directedness is a difficult concept for health care professionals to understand, accept, and implement, it will be much easier for you. It is more consistent with the way you would ordinarily think and behave had you not been so heavily influenced by the health care system. The difficulty you will have is the one you are probably already having: getting what you need from your health care providers.

CHAPTER 6:
Language

Changing paradigms requires changing the language that we use. The following are the words that shape the current problem-oriented medical paradigm. Note: *The definitions are my own and may or may not correspond precisely to those found in dictionaries.*

Words Often Used in Problem-Oriented Care

Normal: Falling within an arbitrary middle range (average) of what is seen in the general population. "Normal" can be used to refer to symptoms, physical findings, physical functions, behaviors, and the results of laboratory and other tests (e.g. X-rays and other imaging studies).

Problem: A detectable abnormality that could potentially result in undesirable symptoms, signs, or other unwanted outcomes.

Symptom: An uncomfortable or worrisome sensation or observation reported by the patient.

Sign: An abnormality detectable by a clinician on physical examination.

Disease: A cluster of abnormal symptoms and/or signs that occur together in a sufficient number of people to warrant a label (e.g., diabetes, rheumatoid arthritis). Diseases tend to have well-established causes, though not always.

Syndrome: A set of two or more symptoms that occur in a sufficient number of people and cause enough discomfort to warrant a label (e.g., restless legs syndrome, dry eyes syndrome). Syndromes tend to be broken up into diseases when the various causes are determined.

Diagnosis: The name given to a disease or syndrome.

Morbidity: A word that once meant the physical and psychological consequences of a disease or syndrome but is now sometimes used interchangeably with "disease" and "syndrome."

Multi-morbidity: More than one disease or syndrome in the same person.

Treatment: The specific remedy for an abnormality.

Management: Measures that may alleviate symptoms and bring signs and test results closer to normal.

Compliance: The degree to which a patient follows the recommendations of the health care team.

Adherence: A slightly less critical-sounding word for compliance.

There are also a number of words and phrases that have been adopted, often by non-physicians, in an attempt to tweak the paradigm. I have already mentioned "palliative care," which is care focused primarily on quality of life and a good death. In a goal-directed health care approach, the term "palliative care" would be redundant and unnecessary. Everyone should get palliative care.

Finally, in a goal-directed paradigm, there would be little or no need for terms like "wholistic medicine" or "complementary and alternative medicine" which refer to care of the whole person and to treatment options that are not usually considered mainstream (like acupuncture, meditation, etc.). As has already been mentioned, non-traditional approaches would probably be considered more often if the focus was on goal-achievement rather than problem-solving. Of course, the strategies recommended by physicians would still have to make sense and be supported by evidence of effectiveness.

Words Used in Goal-Directed Care

The following are some of the new words and phrases required for a goal-directed approach. You may have noticed me using some of these terms in prior chapters. Most are not unique to health care, so they should be familiar. However, you may not have thought very much about their definitions, which are important to this discussion.

Please take the time to read through these terms, and think about how they apply (or don't) to your health and health care experiences.

Goal: A desired outcome that can stand on its own merits. That is, it makes little sense to ask, "Why would you want that to happen?"

Objective: A measurable step along the path to a goal.

Strategy: A way to reach objectives and ultimately a goal. [For example, my 90-year-old mother does balance and leg-strengthening exercises (strategy), in order to be able to walk safely without her walker (objective), so that she can eventually go outside and take care of her plants (goal).]

Obstacle: Anything that gets in the way of the achievement of an objective or goal.

Challenge: A somewhat more positive way to think of an obstacle.

Threshold Principle: The idea that nearly all health challenges are the result of combinations of factors, and that, in each case, a threshold exists above which that combination of factors becomes a significant obstacle to achieving a health goal.

Prioritization: A ranking of strategies based upon their probable impact on goal achievement or a ranking of objectives or goals based upon their importance or achievability.

Premature death: Death resulting from a potentially preventable cause.

Premature disability: Disability resulting from a potentially preventable cause.

Life expectancy: The *average* number of additional years a person or group of people is expected to live.

Health expectancy: The *average* number of additional years a person or group of people is expected to live free of significant disability.

Quality of Life: Your assessment of how great it is to be alive.

Meaningful Life Activity: An activity that gives life joy, purpose, or meaning.

Optimal Growth and Development: 1) Achievement of major developmental tasks; 2) development of resilience, adaptability, and the ability handle challenges; and 3) acquisition of the skills required to help others.

A Good Death: A death that is 1) free from avoidable distress and suffering, for patients, family, and caregivers; 2) in general accord with the patient's and family's wishes; and

3) reasonably consistent with clinical, cultural, and ethical standards.

Same Words, Different Meanings

Finally, some words are useful in both problem-oriented and goal-oriented thinking, but the definitions are somewhat different (as shown in the following table).

WORD	PROBLEM-ORIENTED DEFINITION	GOAL-ORIENTED DEFINITION
Health	A *state* characterized by the absence of physical and psychological abnormalities. Health is viewed as a point on a curve that slopes downward with advancing age.	Making the most one can of life's journey. Health is viewed as the slope of a curve that can be positive, neutral or negative at any age.
Health Care	An applied scientific activity aimed at removing or reducing physical and psychological abnormalities and their consequences.	Strategic relationship-based support intended to help people clarify and achieve their personal health-related goals.
Risk Factor	A characteristic, hazard, or behavior that increases ones risk of an adverse health event. Risk factors for heart attacks include age, gender, increased waist size, inactivity, cigarettes smoking, elevated blood pressure, and high levels of cholesterol in the blood.	A characteristic, hazard, or behavior that reduces ones chance of accomplishing a goal. Risk factors for premature death include increased waist size, inactivity, cigarettes smoking, elevated blood pressure, and high levels of cholesterol in the blood.
Risk Assessment	Documentation and analysis of a person's risk factors to predict and try to prevent the development of health problems.	Analysis of ones risk factors in order to calculate life and health expectancies and determine likely causes of death and disability and obstacles to growth and development and a good death.
Death	A failure of medical care.	Life's final event.

CHAPTER 7:
Who are our Doctors?

"But the person who scored well on an SAT will not necessarily be the best doctor or the best lawyer or the best businessman. These tests do not measure character, leadership, creativity, or perseverance."

—William Julius Wilson

"Too often, educational curricula, instructional methods, and assessment techniques are so tightly constructed that learners have difficulty salvaging the human being – the doctor or the patient – from the educational package in which they are presented."

—Walker Percy, M.D., physician and author

In the late 1980s, Mark Williams and his faculty colleagues at the University of North Carolina Medical School developed a series of innovative modules for training primary care doctors to take better care of older people. The module I found most useful was called "Functional Assessment."

In the video component of the module an elderly man, whose wife has recently died, visits his primary care doctor. The man's vital signs indicate that he has lost a great deal of weight. As he struggles to explain the difficulties he is having with shopping and meal preparation ("I just can't do it the way my Annie did. I miss her so much!"), the doctor reassures him that he can find nothing physically wrong, but that he will order a few tests.

The purpose of the video was to demonstrate the importance of asking about everyday functioning, questions like: "What do you do on a typical day?" and "Are there any things you are having trouble doing?" and "What would you like to be able to do that you can't do now?" The video concludes with a conversation between the main character and a friend about someone they both know who was helped by a physician referral to a physical therapist. Yes, the man was grieving the loss of his wife, but what he needed most was help with shopping and meal preparation.

The premise of the module was straightforward and reasonable—or at least I thought so. But after showing the video to a group of first-year residents, one of them exclaimed, "I didn't go into medicine to be a social worker!"

I was shocked. After regaining my composure, I asked, "Did you go into medicine to help people?" It was the only response I could think of.

Later I realized that there were several reasons the resident responded the way he did. First, he had not been able to identify the patient's functional problem (inability to shop or prepare meals) because he hadn't been taught to ask the right questions. He had also not been taught how to help the patient with those kinds of challenges (what could he do about shopping and cooking troubles) he was facing – so why should he bother trying to identify them? To him, these functional problems were simply white noise drowning out the medical diagnoses he was trained to identify and treat.

Finally, the resident was overwhelmed by the avalanche of biomedical facts that he was being expected to learn. So when he was presented with this hypothetical patient's personal shopping and cooking issues, the resident was essentially thinking, *Do I have to do everything? Where are the social workers?*

What this young man thought he had signed up for when he chose to become a doctor was the challenge of identifying medical problems and prescribing medications and procedures to correct them. He signed up to be an applied scientist: someone who applies scientific knowledge about the human body to correct physical abnormalities.

In the video's final scene, the friend asks the patient, "What did that doctor do for you anyway?" His response is, "Dr. Rusher is a good doctor, but he is looking for serious things."

It turns out that we have trained a generation of doctors (and their patients) to think of diagnosable medical problems as "serious things," and of life's other challenges as somehow less serious or at least not within the purview of physicians.

How are Future Doctors Selected?

The process by which we select future doctors involves two basic steps: (1) a young student's decision to become a doctor and (2) that student's acceptance to medical school. Once someone has been accepted to medical school, they nearly always complete their training.

Who in your high school class did teachers and counselors advise to consider a career in medicine? I suspect it was those with good grades who were especially good at math and science. Why was that?

I think it is because medicine is viewed as an applied science. As such, university prerequisites for medical school are mostly science courses. While many medical schools encourage a well-rounded education, courses in the social sciences and humanities are rarely considered essential.

But health care should be about so much more than the application of science to the treatment of human diseases. Health care, at its core, is about *caring for and about people.*

Our educational system ought to be encouraging altruistic students with excellent interpersonal skills to become doctors. And we should insist that those math-and-science whiz-kids be exposed to the social sciences and humanities, because they will need that knowledge to provide high quality care to their future patients.

There are many reasons people choose medicine as a career. Some do it because of family expectations, others because it is a relatively lucrative, recession-proof career. For some, medicine is an alternative to becoming a researcher or university professor.

And some—hopefully many—are truly interested in serving others. It is this population of doctors that we should be identifying and encouraging. Students who are exceptional in math and science are already being identified and encouraged. We should look harder for those whose gifts include interpersonal skills, judgment, and emotional maturity.

The Medical School Admission Process

Medical school admission committees are faced with many more qualified applicants than positions. All applicants have high grade point averages and long lists of extracurricular activities. For that reason, admission committees rely heavily on Medical College Admissions Test (MCAT) scores and personal interviews.

The MCAT has evolved from a test of knowledge, primarily in math and science, to the ability to apply scientific knowledge to solve problems. One of the four sections of the test does focus on the social sciences and humanities. Nearly all applicants have taken an MCAT prep course. Applicants meeting the MCAT cutoff are interviewed by doctors, most of whom view medicine as an applied science. The result is predictable.

Of course we want doctors to understand science. And being a good science student is very helpful during the first two years of medical school, which are filled with science courses. However, things begin to change when students reach the final two years of medical school, when interpersonal skills become more important. That is when students must decide how much they enjoy interactions. Many areas of medicine require very little human contact with patients (e.g., radiology, anesthesiology, pathology, many of the procedural specialties, and basic research).

Be sure to thank doctors who have chosen to provide direct care for patients. They have often chosen to do so despite that fact that they could have made more money and had more predictable hours had they chosen a different specialty.

How Doctors are Trained

Doctors must complete college, then four years of medical school, followed by at least three of residency, and sometimes one to three years of fellowship. Each of these steps is designed to draw students and trainees progressively into the world and culture of medicine.

When I entered medical school, I was given a test to determine my baseline medical knowledge. I had to guess at the answers to most of the questions because I didn't understand them. When I took the same test at the end of medical school, it struck me that the most important keys to success on the test were a new vocabulary and a way of thinking.

Medical School

Typically, the coursework in the first two years of medical school includes normal anatomy, biochemistry, physiology, and psychology, followed by the study of the abnormalities that can occur in each of those areas. It is often organized by organ system (e.g. digestive system, neurological system, urinary system, etc.). Some of this material is taught using a technique called *problem-based learning*, in which students work together in small groups to solve clinical problems within the context of cases.

Most medical schools include a course on patient interviewing and physical examination skills. Depending upon who teaches it, there may be some or even a great deal of emphasis on communication skills. Some medical schools train laypeople to act as simulated patients. If you live near a medical school, consider signing up to be a simulated patient. These early courses are sometimes the only time during the entire medical school curriculum when students are encouraged to learn something about their patients as human beings.

During the third and fourth years of medical school, students rotate through a series of specialty services, mostly in the hospital setting. Clinical knowledge and skills are taught by residents, who are in turn supervised by faculty. During a series of 4 to 6-week rotations, students hone their abilities to take a problem-focused history, perform a physical examination, formulate a list of possible diagnoses, order the correct tests and consultations, make a presumptive diagnosis, and generate a treatment plan. By the mid-point of their fourth year in medical school, students must choose a medical specialty in which to continue their training.

Medical school tuition varies from around $30,000 to $60,000 per year. The average debt incurred by students by the time of graduation is now more than $200,000. That level of debt often influences graduates to choose specialties with higher average incomes, which will allow them to pay their debts off more quickly. It is an incentive for students to choose the procedural specialties over interpersonal specialties like primary care.

Residency and Fellowship

Most physicians complete at least three years of residency training after medical school, some as many as seven. Most of this training, even in the primary care fields of family medicine, general internal medicine, and pediatrics, occurs in hospitals. Some non-surgical specialties like endocrinology, rheumatology, gastroenterology, and neonatology require an additional one to three years of fellowship. Fellowships typically include at least one year of research training.

During residency doctors begin to take responsibility for the care of patients. Their first priority is to learn how to handle the avalanche of administrative work (i.e., notes, orders, prescriptions, referrals, visit summaries, discharge summaries, etc.) required to make the system work efficiently. Their other concern is to learn how to handle life-threatening emergencies (e.g., cardiac arrest, hemorrhage, etc.).

Once those things have been mastered, these doctors-in-training can focus on their diagnostic skills. Because efficiency is essential, they learn to ask just enough questions and do just enough physical examination to decide which tests to order. Their hope (and assumption) is that most conditions can be diagnosed using the many tests now available. And they soon figure out that, once they make the correct diagnosis, management instructions can be found on their computers in online programs like Up-to-Date.

The over-reliance on testing and the under-appreciation of the value of a carful history and examination is a recent phenomenon, which has almost certainly contributed to the rising cost of health care. Just a few extra minutes of well-spent time with patients would reduce the number of unnecessary, expensive, and sometimes hazardous tests. A particular patient comes to mind.

Mrs. Spencer was a 60 year-old woman who, while returning from a vacation, had a heart rhythm disturbance severe enough to require emergency room treatment. The emergency room physician advised her to see me when she got home, which she did. I reviewed her personal history, the circumstances surrounding the event, and her medical history. She reported some mild, intermittent asthma and had had a hysterectomy 15 years earlier. During my physical examination, I noticed a scar at the base of her neck. She recalled that prior to her hysterectomy she had had an abnormal chest X-ray, which led to a biopsy of some lymph nodes in her chest. They had told her there was evidence of sarcoidosis, but they reassured her that nothing further needed to be done since it was asymptomatic. My suspicion of cardiac sarcoidosis as the cause of her rhythm disturbance was subsequently confirmed by specific tests. Treatment was successful and most likely life-saving

By the time residents reach their third year, they are so firmly entrenched in a problem-oriented approach that it is virtually impossible to retrain them. The primary objective for most residents at that point is to finish their training and find a job.

Many residents with whom I have worked acknowledge the potential advantages of a goal-directed approach. They agree that the health care system is broken, but they have become so good at problem solving that they really don't want to think about having to learn a whole new way of thinking and acting.

Training Sites

Hospitals have never been good places to train doctors. This was pointed out by Sir Francis Peabody in a 1927 article published in the Journal of the American Medical Association. "Hospitals, like other institutions founded with the highest human ideals, are apt to deteriorate into dehumanizing machines, and even the physician who has the patient's welfare most at heart finds the pressure of work forces him to give most of his attention to the critically sick and to those whose diseases that are a menace to the public health.

In such cases he must first treat the specific disease, and there then remains little time in which to cultivate more than a superficial personal contact with the patients."

Since Dr. Peabody's time the situation has only gotten worse. The discovery that keeping patients in bed was a bad idea reduced hospital lengths of stay dramatically in the 1970s. Then, as a result of cost-cutting measures (e.g., payment of hospitals based upon patients' diagnoses instituted in 1983), there was a financial incentive for hospitals to keep lengths of stay short.

In addition, most hospital emergency rooms are now staffed by contract physicians who are incentivized to see lots of patients and avoid liability. That has a tendency to result in the admission of patients who wouldn't have needed hospital-ization if someone had more time to evaluate them or if the physician evaluating them knew them better. Consequently, the average length of stay for most hospitalized patients is only 2 or 3 days.

Because patients don't stay in the hospital very long, the trainees rarely have sufficient time to get to know much about them. Worse, because of the revolving door nature of hospitals these days, the medical trainees end up spending a majority of their time on the extensive documentation involved in admitting and discharging patients.

Attending (i.e. faculty) physicians generally rotate through the hospital teaching service for one to four weeks at a time. In addition to teaching, their responsibilities include making sure that residents don't make serious mistakes, that all paperwork is properly completed and signed, that billing information is correctly forwarded, and that the patients get admitted and discharged in a timely manner. That leaves little time to spend with patients or for bedside teaching. Discussions on teaching rounds therefore tend to focus on patients' current medical conditions, diagnostic evaluations, consultant recommendations, treatment options, and discharge plans.

Residents in training do spend time in outpatient settings, but, in most residency programs, this tends to be focused on one-time hospital follow-up visits. The exception is the primary care residencies in which trainees spend up to 4 half-days per week in the clinic taking care of their own patients over time. Most primary care residents also spend time in nursing homes and assisted living settings, and they even receive a little bit of training in how to make home visits.

An Alternative

In terms of content, there is no compelling reason why the medical school curriculum could not be organized around a combination of life stages and the four major health care goals. Placing our knowledge of how the body works within a lifespan framework would make it possible to emphasize the changes that occur at various phases of life. The focus on goals would help students understand how and when that knowledge might apply to people, and it would make it possible to emphasize the existence and importance of human diversity.

There is also no reason why the core didactic courses have to be clustered within the first two years of medical school. Students would probably benefit more from working directly with patients from the beginning and throughout the entire curriculum. Problem-based learning modules are a step in that direction, and that concept could easily be refocused on patient goals rather than on problem-solving. It would simply require an additional source of information, a (simulated) patient to answer person-centered questions from the students. Students could also be assigned to a small panel of patients they could follow throughout the four years. In fact, something similar is already being done in some medical schools now.

While all students regardless of ultimate career path would need the proposed goal-directed curriculum, some differentiation could, and probably should, occur during the final portion of the curriculum. Students destined to become primary care physicians - family physicians, pediatricians, and general internists – would need more advanced and expanded training in goal-directed care while future subspecialists could spend additional time on subjects of particular relevance to them. For example, future surgeons might wish to spend more time studying anatomy.

There are many possible solutions to the student debt problem. One which appears to have worked fairly well is debt forgiveness for students who complete a residency in a primary care specialty and then practice for a specified period of time in a community that needs primary care physicians.

If medical students received the sort of education and training I am proposing, it would be easier to design goal-directed primary care residency experiences. The biggest obstacles would be faculty retraining and development of training sites. Fortunately, since much of the teaching that goes on in residencies occurs between upper level residents and lower level residents, universal buy-in by and retraining of primary care faculty might not be essential. As long as the faculty responsible for organizing the curriculum and those who evaluate and certify residency programs are on board, goal-directed training of primary care residents should be possible.

Aside from a reorientation of the curriculum around goals, the most critical aspect of primary care residency training is the settings in which training occurs. Teaching settings for primary care clinicians should reflect the settings in which they will be practicing. The practice of goal-directed care would involve a somewhat different professional team, which I will discuss further in a subsequent chapter, and it would require an even greater emphasis on continuity of care – taking care of the same group of patients and families over time. Time spent in hospitals should be reduced, and time spent in patients homes increased.

Goal-oriented concepts should be included in subspecialty residency curricula as well, but to a much lesser degree. The most important lessons subspecialists need to learn are the importance of longitudinal primary care relationships and the importance of knowing the difference between what can be done and what should be done for a particular patient.

The Medical Hierarchy

In most large corporations, there is a Chief Executive Officer (CEO) who is expected to direct and coordinate the activities of the entire organization. To be effective, that person must have broad knowledge of how the different parts of the company fit together. They must focus on the goals of the enterprise and instill organizational values. CEOs are mission-driven, goal-oriented generalists, and the people working in each department or division of the organization are akin to the subspecialists of the health care system. The CEO has ultimate authority and responsibility and, therefore, earns the highest salary.

Within the current health care system, the opposite is true. Subspecialists have greater status and authority and earn much higher salaries than primary care doctors (generalists). This is, to a large degree, a natural consequence of the problem-oriented medical paradigm, in which doctors who know the most about diseases are awarded the highest status.

Subspecialists are, and should be, problem-solvers. A physician who specializes in gastrointestinal diseases – a gastroenterologist - must be adept at identifying and treating diseases of the stomach and intestines. A neurologist must know more than anyone else about diseases of the brain and nervous system. A cardiothoracic surgeon must be able to surgically correct abnormalities of the heart, lungs and blood vessels.

But, just as businesses need CEOs, the health care system works best when someone is coordinating each person's care and paying attention to the mission of the system and the goals of individual patients. Otherwise there is a significant probability that irrelevant problems will be discovered and treated, costing the system, and therefore all of us, lots of money and causing patients unnecessary harm.

The subspecialist-dominant medical hierarchy is therefore a major obstacle to the adoption of goal-directed health care. Academic medical centers have traditionally been the place where people with the most complex health problems are sent. It isn't surprising then that academic hospitals are filled with subspecialists and super-subspecialists (e.g. neurologists that only treat children with seizures). But those doctors have become, by force of numbers, the dominant decision-makers when it comes to establishing medical school prerequisites, admission criteria, and curricula. While primary care doctors are present, they are in the minority.

The result is that *all* medical students are taught to think like subspecialists. The basic science courses are taught by research scientists with narrow areas of knowledge and expertise. A majority of the 4 to 8-week clinical rotations are focused on learning about the problems that define each subspecialty. The various subspecialty departments fight for space in the curriculum because clinical rotations are also used to recruit students into residency programs.

To make matters worse, many subspecialty faculty members have a negative opinion - based upon a limited understanding - of primary care and try to dissuade the best students from choosing it as a career path. When speaking with a top medical student, they might say something like: "You would be wasting your brain if you become a primary care physician. All they see each day are runny noses and sore throats." The same subspecialist is just as likely to say: "It is impossible to do primary care well. There is far too much to learn."

In other words, primary care is both too easy *and* too hard.

This apparent contradiction arises from the fact that the appropriate focus of primary care is on people and processes (making the health care system work for their patients) rather than on diseases (more on this later). For that reason, when primary care doctors are involved in consultations and referrals, things generally go better for patients. When that doesn't happen, patients can get swept up in a cascade of unnecessary tests and treatments.

Outside of academic centers, the hierarchy is less pronounced but still important. In that setting, subspecialists are more dependent on referrals from primary care doctors, so they are more likely to be supportive. Informal phone and hallway consultations between generalists and subspecialists are more common. Primary care physicians have a bit more influence over the course of events, but the income disparities still create tension.

Income Inequality

The large difference in income between subspecialists and primary care physicians is an important barrier to the adoption of goal-directed care. Largely because of the subspecialist-dominated medical hierarchy, procedures are reimbursed (e.g., by Medicare, Medicaid, and private insurance companies) at a higher rate than time spent talking, listening, and reasoning. As a result, subspecialists who perform procedures (e.g., surgeons, gastroenterologists, and cardiologists) earn significantly more than primary care doctors.

Primary care doctors have tended to react to the income differences by seeing more patients and trying to do more procedures. Some reduce the number of older and more complex patients they accept, and they are quicker to refer patients with more significant medical conditions. These strategies ensure that they see a higher percentage of patients with simple problems. A primary care physician who sees six patients with sore throats in an hour will generate more income than one who sees two elderly patients with multiple chronic health-impacting challenges.

The subspecialty-dominant medical hierarchy is reinforced by the media. It is the dramatic procedures (e.g., face and hand transplants, gene therapy, prenatal heart surgery, etc.) that make the best news, even though they will only ever benefit a very small number of people. Helping ordinary people live longer, enjoy life a bit more, become wiser and more resilient, and experience good deaths is nowhere near as exciting.

CHAPTER 8:

Record Keeping, Billing, and Reimbursement

"You don't train someone for all of those years of medical school and residency, particularly people who want to help others optimize their physical and psychological health, and then have them run a claims-processing operation for insurance companies."

—*Malcolm Gladwell*

I recently scheduled an appointment with my primary care doctor using the internet "portal" that is connected to his practice's electronic medical record. I was asked to answer a series of questions in preparation for the visit. There was a page of questions about medical problems I may have had, a page of questions about past surgical procedures, and a third page about medical problems that run in my family.

On the final page of the questionnaire there was a single question about me, the person. It asked, "Please tell us who lives with you and any other pertinent information about yourself." I wrote, "I live with my wife, Sandy, and my golden retriever, Lily. I…"

At that point I ran out of space, so I deleted the "I."

There were no questions about meaningful life activities, advance directives, resources, limitations, or personal values. I was curious to see how the tidbit of personal information I was able to provide was handled in the record, so I went back online to find it.

And it was gone. (I'm sure it is still in there somewhere, but it was not visible or editable by me.)

A Short History of Modern Medical Records

Prior to 1975 the records kept by most doctors consisted of an initial, complete medical history with the following sections:

History of the present illness (main health concerns today)

Past medical history (health problems in the past that are no longer active)

Social history (marital status, living situation, education and occupation, racial/ethnic identification, religion, hobbies, sexual orientation, and unhealthy behaviors)

Family medical history "(potentially hereditary health conditions experienced by close family members).

Review of systems (a catch-all list of symptoms the patient might have forgotten to mention)

Physical examination followed by an assessment (current diagnoses) and plan (mostly current medications and other planned treatments).

Subsequent visit notes were short phrases without subheadings documenting new findings and actions taken. When I was a medical student, it wasn't at all uncommon for medical records of general practitioners in the community to be kept on 3" by 5" index cards. A typical visit note might have look liked this.

"Strep throat. Penicillin VK 250mg QID for 10 days."

In 1964, Lawrence Weed, a primary care doctor from Vermont, pointed out the weaknesses in this approach, and in anticipation of computerization, he suggested a new method of record keeping that he called the "problem-oriented medical record." He recommended that the initial evaluation note begin with a "Patient Profile," which would take the place of the social history and be enriched over time. The rest of the initial note was similar to traditional evaluation notes, except that the "History of Present Illness" included a separate paragraph for each problem.

He suggested that progress notes be organized into the individual problems addressed at the visit, with each problem section divided into four parts: (1) subjective information obtained from the patient, (2) objective information from examination and testing, (3) assessment, and (4) plans for treatment and follow-up. Finally, he suggested that every record include a "Problem List" comprised of all of the active health problems identified in that individual.

Weed's ideas began to take hold in the early 1970's, and many of them have been universally adopted by clinicians, insurance companies, and electronic health records vendors. The problem-oriented medical record was adopted because it was a better representation of the way physicians had learned to think. It reflected the rapid advancement of the science of diseases and their treatment. Unfortunately, some of Weed's better ideas, such as placing a personal description of the patient and their interests at the beginning of the evaluation note, were largely ignored.

Despite all of the touted benefits of computerization, the health care system was one of the last industries to embrace and adopt computer technologies. Electronic medical records have been available since the 1970s, but, as recently as ten years ago only a small minority of physicians and hospitals used them. Finally, in an all-out effort to improve coordination of care and reduce costs, the federal government made electronic health record implementation a priority. Significant financial incentives were paid to physicians and hospitals through both Medicare and Medicaid to help with the cost of conversion from paper to electronic records. As of January 2015, all doctors have had to use electronic medical records to avoid financial penalties.

Virtually all electronic medical record systems are problem-oriented. All have a "Problem List." All have a "Disposition" section that requires labeling and coding of each problem dealt with at the visit. Everything that can possibly be is numerically coded. Visit notes are, for the most part, created by clicking boxes in pre-coded templates.

As a result, modern EMR's are mechanical and impersonal. Only a few display any sort of personal information on their opening page. In most cases, that information is buried in the Social History section, which can only be accessed by clicking several buttons … rather than being the first thing that the physician sees when opening your record.

The Evolving Purpose of Medical Records

Prior to 1985, the main purpose of medical records was to document clinical information useful to the care of patients. Payment for medical services was based upon the concept of "customary, prevailing, and reasonable rates," largely determined by the physician based upon time spent with the patient. As the number of medical malpractice lawsuits increased during the second half of the twentieth century, somewhat better documentation became necessary, and notes became a bit longer, but their primary purpose remained clinical care.

However, since 1985, Medicare has made several significant changes in the way the value of physicians' services is calculated, and Medicaid and the private insurance companies followed suit. Those changes required even more detailed documentation, so detailed in fact that many physicians accept lower fees rather than spending the time on the documentation required to charge appropriately.

This challenge provided a window of opportunity for the developers of electronic medical records. Physicians otherwise reluctant to purchase an expensive electronic record system could be convinced that the record would pay for itself by making the documentation required for higher reimbursement rates easier. That marketing strategy resulted in the development of electronic medical records designed primarily for the optimization of billing and reimbursement. The ability to generate preprogrammed verbage by pushing a button on the computer has resulted in notes that are so long and redundant that, once created, they are hardly ever read again (except by auditors).

And despite the promise of greater efficiency and higher reimbursement rates, most primary care physicians have found that the amount of time spent on documentation has actually added a significant amount of additional work. Many have had to reduce the number of patients they see each day, and they still have to work through lunch and into the evening just to complete their records. And both physicians and patients complain that the computer interferes with person-to-person interactions during visits.

Impact of Current Medical Record Systems on Goal-Directed Care

The electronic medical records in use today are one of the greatest obstacles to the adoption and implementation of goal-directed health care. The most prominent sections in all electronic medical records are the Problem List and the Medication List. Those two sections are tightly linked to the Assessment and Plan sections of each visit note. Disease-oriented templates remind physicians and their staff of what questions to ask and which examinations to perform for each problem, turning mouse clicks into text.

The least prominent and least used section is the Social History, which is generally relegated to a free-text form pulled forward into visit notes for reimbursement purposes. It is most often used to document behavioral problems like use of tobacco and alcohol. Forms are available for recording functional status (i.e. problems carrying out daily activities), but they are rarely used, and it is even less common to find information about activities the patient values or wants to be able to do. There is no section for patient goals.

While most systems provide reminders of preventive services for which each patient is eligible, none of which I am aware prioritize those services with regard to projected impact on that person's length of life. There is usually a small section in which to indicate whether the patient has an advance directive, but the conditions under which they would no longer wish to be kept alive and preferences for end-of-life care are practically never recorded. Only pediatric records include forms on which to document personal development, and they generally only include standard developmental milestones.

A major disadvantage of current electronic medical records is that they break a person's health story into individual encounters, making it difficult to see patterns over time or to understand the longitudinal context in which events have occurred. Paper records weren't much better in this regard, but it would have been much easier to modify them. In other words electronic record systems have served to cement in place the problem-oriented medical model for years to come.

Finally, despite the provisions in the Health Information Privacy and Portability Act (HIPPA) and the requirements for "Meaningful Use of Electronic Medical Records," most current electronic record systems are not truly interactional. That is, you may be able to look at parts of your record online, submit questions to your doctor, and enter some medical information on standard forms, but you cannot do much to make your record your own. If you want a record that actually helps you to achieve your personal health goals, you will have to create a separate "Personal Health Record." And while a number of companies are now marketing such products, most are still based upon traditional problem-oriented thinking.

A goal-directed health record would be organized around the major goals of health and health care with sections for risk assessment, prioritization of preventive services, and conditions worse than death; functional assessments and documentation of meaningful life activities; developmental milestones, personal growth and resilience, and relational skills; and advance directives and values and preferences regarding end-of-life care. Each section would include periodic reevaluations of goals, strategies, and progress and timelines on which to view progress and recalculations.

Health challenges (e.g. discovery of ovarian cancer) would be linked to the goal areas to which they pertained.

Billing and Reimbursement

It has always been difficult for Medicare, Medicaid, and private health insurance companies to quantify (that is, figure out how much money they should pay for) medical care that does not involve a specific procedure, such as a surgical operation, X-ray, laboratory test, etc. How valuable is the application of knowledge, wisdom, and judgment? What about the time required to establish relationships with patients? What about the time spent reviewing medical records from previous physicians or the time, effort, and expertise involved in coordinating care among the various consultants and services? And how can those kinds of activities be documented without taking time away from the time spent providing the care?

I vividly remember, during my first years in private practice, successfully resuscitating a man in our office and spending the next hour keeping him alive until the cardiologists at the hospital could take over. He had had a heart attack, which cause his heart to stop right in my examination room. It was a Saturday, and our staff was new and unfamiliar with our resuscitation equipment. The small town rescue squad neglected to bring a defibrillator when they arrived at the office, and the EKG monitor in their ambulance didn't work. On the way to the hospital, 20 minutes away, I kept talking to him with my finger on the pulse in his wrist. When he stopped talking and his pulse disappeared, I shocked him back to life. That happened at least four times.

When I finally got back home, covered in blood and vomit, totally exhausted, my wife remembers me asking her how much she thought I should charge. She says I asked if $100 would be too much. (Remember, this was 1979.)

I saw that same man, who was not a regular patient of ours, in the office for a minor illness a year later. I don't think he remembered who I was. After all, he wasn't himself that day. I don't remember what we ended up charging him for saving his life. He didn't complain about it, and I never worried that someone from Medicare would audit my records and make me pay them back.

In those days, in the late 1970s, the insurance companies generally trusted physicians to charge appropriately, and the vast majority of us did. However, a small proportion did purposely over-charge, and, rather than seeking out and punishing those few, the federal government decided to make it more difficult for physicians to cheat.

Thus, in an attempt to tighten up the billing process, in 1985, the Centers for Medicare and Medicaid Services commissioned the development of a new reimbursement system based upon a complicated formula that included the physical effort, skill required, malpractice risk, and complexity involved in each patient encounter. However, no actual data existed upon which to determine those factors and so it didn't work very well.

In 1992, the algorithm was modified to include documentation of physician work (questions asked, diagnoses made, treatments prescribed), practice expense (estimated as an average by a special panel of physicians) and cost of malpractice insurance (average for the specialty of the physician). The physician work component accounted for 48% of the total. This modification was called Evaluation and Management (E&M) Coding, and it was, of course, based on the problem-oriented medical model.

The Evaluation and Management Approach

E&M coding is a points-based system. For each doctor-patient interaction, points are awarded for each appropriate question asked by the doctor (history taking), each part of the physical examination completed, and the complexity of the visit as determined by the number of problems managed, lab tests ordered, and prescriptions written (decision-making). The total "value" of each visit is based upon a complicated sum of the items in each of those categories, multiplied by a factor that takes into account years of training and risk of liability. In order to submit a bill to Medicare, at least one and no more than four diagnoses must be listed by code number on the billing form. Medicaid and most private insurance companies have adopted this billing method, but each payer has their own unique forms.

Aside from being more complicated and probably no more accurate than the previous method, E&M coding effectively locks doctors into a problem-oriented approach. They are financially rewarded for identifying a problem, determining the cause, and prescribing a treatment, and not for very much else. The point system applies best when the patient has a set of symptoms, and the object is to determine the cause of those symptoms and prescribe a medication or procedure.

In my geriatric practice, most visits were not like that at all. About 90% of visits involved conversations, and most often those conversations involved figuring out how to help patients function better. Physical examination was only occasionally helpful for any purpose other than reassurance. (Note: When your physician examines your heart and lungs even when your concerns are completely unrelated to those systems, it is most likely an attempt to get more bullet points for billing purposes.) While I was always able to come up with a list of "diagnoses" for billing purposes, that list rarely captured what actually happened during the visit.

Many physicians, myself included, refused to memorize the complex E&M rules and simply undercharged to avoid trouble. Others hired additional staff to calculate the correct billing codes, while still others bought electronic medical record systems that would do the calculation for them automatically.

Newer Approaches

The E&M coding and billing method was created for use in a fee-for-service delivery model, which has been the predominant payment model for medical services throughout history. Fee-for-service simply means that patients are charged for each visit separately, based upon the services that were performed. However, economists have pointed out that the fee-for-service approach incentivizes doctors to provide more services, recommend more visits, order more tests, and do more procedures. They argue that fee-for-service is one of the most important drivers of our increasing health care costs.

In the 1980s, many Medicaid programs and some commercial insurers instituted a radically different payment process called "managed care." In a managed care model, primary care physicians are paid a set amount of money per patient per month, and they are then expected to provide them with comprehensive and coordinated care. A certain percentage of the payments are withheld and are paid, along with a percentage of any savings accrued, at the end of each year if the cost of care has been less than projected.

Because these end-of-year payments are based upon the total cost of care for these patients, including the care provided by subspecialists and hospitals, primary care physicians are financially incentivized to reduce the use of expensive treatments and procedures, referrals and consultations, and hospitalizations. That puts primary care physicians in the role of "gatekeepers," a role which they at first welcomed but soon rejected as they found themselves trying to talk patients out of requested services and wondering if they were doing so for financial or valid medical reasons. Despite this potential conflict of interest, some managed care plans have survived (e.g., Kaiser Permanente), but most were abandoned in favor of a return to fee-for-service or some combination of fee-for-service and managed care.

Passage of the Patient Protection and Affordable Care Act in 2010 established the Centers for Medicare and Medicaid

Innovations (CMMI), the mission of which is to improve the quality and effectiveness of health care while reducing its cost. A number of important experiments have been conducted or are underway, all of which involve new payment models. The two approaches that appear to have gained the most traction to date are "accountable care organizations" (ACOs) and "value-based purchasing."

Value-based purchasing ties reimbursement rates to both cost and quality of care. There is often a component of fee-for-service reimbursement in addition to a value-based component. Accountable care organizations are essentially managed care organizations that fund and hold accountable an entire system of doctors and hospitals rather than individual physicians. In addition, like value-based purchasing models, they base financial incentives on both cost containment and quality of care.

By adding the quality of care component, these models attempt to reduce the impact of the still-present conflict of interest created by tying financial gain to medical decisions. That strategy rests on the very questionable assumption that value can be fairly and accurately measured using current problem-oriented metrics. It assumes, for example, that nearly everyone with an elevated blood pressure needs, and wants, and has the resources necessary to bring their blood pressure down. It also assumes that blood pressure reduction is a reliable measure of the quality of care delivered by clinicians regardless of their patient population. But that simply isn't true.

For example, a doctor with an upper middle class, well-educated suburban practice, who is really good at getting patients' blood pressure under control regardless of whether it was helpful to do so in all cases, would be credited with providing high quality care. On the other hand, a doctor working in a free clinic in which most patients are unable to afford medications, a high proportion are addicted to alcohol or have serious mental illnesses, and most would benefit very little from attempts to lower their blood pressure, would receive lower quality scores and less reimbursement.

Goal-directed health care would function best if health care was viewed as a public good rather than a commodity, the assumption being that our society is stronger when we are all healthy. It seems to me that primary care should be exempted from the reimbursement schemes discussed above. Since primary care isn't particularly expensive – some have estimated its cost at around $25 to $50 per patient per month – state or federal pools could be created to pay primary care physicians on a salaried basis with incentives based not on numbers of patients seen, above reasonable minimums, but on the quality of care provided, based upon patient-oriented outcome measures. Salaries would need to be high enough to make it attractive and financially feasible for medical students to choose a career in primary care despite their student debts.

CHAPTER 9:
Clinical Practice Guidelines

"Whereas in times past the 'right thing' was an ethical construct enshrined in the values of the caregiving professions, it is now a particular drug, test, or strategy supported by the burgeoning medical literature."

—Richard M.J. Bohmer

"The unbridled enthusiasm for guidelines, and the unrealistic expectations about what they will accomplish, frequently betrays inexperience and unfamiliarity with their limitations and potential hazards."

—Steven H. Woolf, MD, PhD and colleagues

Clinical Practice Guidelines and Problem-Oriented Care

In the late 1980s, a series of studies conducted by Wennberg at Dartmouth showed wide geographic variation in the rates of performance of many expensive medical procedures.

Those discoveries and advances in scientific and statistical methods contributed to the birth of "evidence-based medicine," which is defined as "the conscientious, explicit, and judicious use of current best evidence in making decisions about the care of individual patients."

Again you are probably wondering, "Haven't doctors always based their recommendations upon the best available scientific evidence?" The answer is a qualified no. Doctors have, of course, always used their best "judgment," which can be defined as a combination of what they were taught in school, what they learned from refresher courses and journals, and their own clinical experience. As you might expect, when faced with the same information, this approach could lead different doctors to different conclusions.

The evidence-based medicine movement was and is an attempt to encourage physicians to rely more heavily on the results of research, which is believed to reduce variability and lead to better overall care for the majority of patients. Using advanced statistical methods, researchers are able to combine and summarize the results of multiple studies. These "systematic reviews" and "meta-analyses" can then be used to develop recommendations called "clinical practice guidelines." Clinical practice guidelines are intended to turn mountains of research findings into practice advice for health care professionals. They were never intended to be rigid or binding on clinicians or patients. However, as payments to clinicians are increasingly based upon the "value" (quality of care divided by cost) of services provided, guidelines have morphed into the standards of care upon which doctors are evaluated and paid.

Guidelines are viewed by payers (e.g., Medicare/Medicaid and private insurance companies) as a way to incorporate marketplace principles into health care, in order to bring down costs. Their hope is that people will choose health care services based upon quality as measured by conformance to the guidelines, and that guideline-based care will be less expensive. Many reinforce guideline adherence by rewarding or penalizing doctors, based upon whether they meet quality standards derived from the guidelines.

For example, a doctor could receive a bonus if more than 75% of her eligible female patients have received a pap smear. Or that doctor could be penalized financially if the percentage of their patients with average blood sugar levels below 170 is lower than 80%.

At this point, you should be able to see how clinical practice guidelines reinforce the problem-oriented approach. First, they begin and end with disease identification and management. Goals, as we have defined them, are rarely mentioned. Second, there is usually no effort to quantify the benefits of the recommendations making it difficult for physicians to base their recommendations on the unique goals and challenges of individual patients.

The quality measures derived from guidelines generally assume that every person should be treated the same way (e.g., everyone should have a blood pressure of less than 140/80). This is an industrial model of quality assurance in which the objective is to make sure that every widget meets the same specifications.

In stark contrast, the goal-directed approach begins with the assumption that every person is different and should therefore be treated differently. Keeping average blood pressure below 140/90 is more important for some people than for others, and, for some people, blood pressure control is unnecessary and irrelevant.

An example of a widely accepted guideline recommendation taken from the American Diabetes Association's (ADA) Type 2 Diabetes Guideline is as follows:

"Lowering A1c to approximately 7% [an average blood sugar of 154] or less has been shown to reduce microvascular complications [blindness, kidney failure, nerve damage] of diabetes and, if implemented soon after the diagnosis of diabetes, is associated with long-term reduction in macrovascular [heart attacks, strokes] disease. Therefore, a reasonable A1c goal for many non-pregnant adults is less than 7%. (B)"

[Note: Because I mentioned it earlier, I will again point out that there is no evidence that lowering blood sugar in people with Type 2 (adult-onset) diabetes has any appreciable effect on the rate of heart attacks and strokes though certain diabetes medications may lower risk somewhat through other mechanisms. The evidence used to make the argument in the Type 2 diabetes guideline was based primarily upon studies of people with Type 1 diabetes, a completely different disease.]

Clues that this recommendation came from a disease-oriented guideline are:

The outcomes mentioned - microvascular and macrovascular complications - are disease-oriented outcomes. No information is provided about whether lowering blood sugar levels would increase length or quality of life or any specific area of function or type of activity. Interestingly, the well-documented benefit of lowering blood sugar on symptom reduction is not mentioned.

There is also no indication of the size of the effect of lowering blood sugar levels on any meaningful outcomes.

Finally, no attempt is made to point out whether other factors like physical activity, blood pressure, cholesterol level, tobacco use could be expected to increase or reduce the hazards of high blood sugar levels, potentially modifying the need for aggressive treatment.

Since each guideline is developed independently, the guidelines for different diseases don't always mesh. In 2005, Cynthia Boyd and her colleagues at Johns Hopkins published a paper in the Journal of the American Medical Association showing what would happen if a patient with emphysema, high blood pressure, diabetes, osteoporosis, and arthritis (all very common conditions in the elderly) followed the guidelines for each of those conditions. Such a patient would need to take 12 different medicines, costing more than $400 per month, on a very complicated schedule, risking a number of drug-to-drug interactions.

And because guidelines focus on individual diseases, they seem to contribute to fragmented thinking on the part of physicians.

While teaching at a local nursing home, I met a woman I will call Jane. Jane had recently been discharged from the hospital after a three-week stay during which she almost died from disturbances of her blood chemistries, kidney failure, confusion and hallucinations, anemia (low red blood cell counts), and malnutrition. This last admission was the longest of a series of hospitalizations over the prior year for similar problems. Upon reviewing all of her hospital discharge summaries, it was clear that she had received excellent disease-oriented care. Every individual abnormality had been addressed. At the time of discharge her lab test results were as good as they were ever going to be.

Very little information was available from Jane's records about who she was as a person or how she came to be so sick again and again. However, buried within her Social History was a mention of occasional heavy alcohol use, which seemed like it might be important in view of her many medical challenges. I decided, with her permission, to sit down and talk with her and her two daughters.

During our conversation Jane and her daughters revealed that, over the past year, Jane had lived with a long-time boyfriend who she acknowledged was an alcoholic. Her daughters reported that since she had been living with the boyfriend she had also been drinking heavily. They believed that she would be unable to quit drinking as long as she was in that environment.

I told Jane in the presence of her sisters that if she continued to drink heavily she would almost certainly end up back in the hospital, and the next time she could very easily die. I emphasized the point by asking her to consider all the reasons she had for wanting to stay alive. Jane was clearly not ready to die. She reluctantly agreed that she wouldn't be able to stop drinking as long as she was living with the boyfriend. One of the daughters invited her to live with her, and she decided to try it, at least for awhile.

Jane subsequently became my patient. She did not return to the boyfriend and was able to quit drinking. As a result, she did well for a number of years until her kidneys eventually failed, requiring dialysis.

In theory, Jane might have done just as well with disease-oriented care if her most important disease, alcoholism, had been identified. However, the doctors who had taken care of her had become distracted by all of her individual problems, the ones that were more obvious because they produced abnormal laboratory test results. But by focusing on the goal, survival, I was able to zero in on her alcohol abuse, and I was able to clarify the situation for her and her daughters in a way that helped the three of them develop effective strategies.

Clinical Practice Guidelines and Electronic Registries

You may have already received a phone call or e-mail message similar to the following. (If not, you probably will.)

Dear Ms. Smith:

We regularly review our records to make sure that we have advised all of our patients about preventive services that might benefit them. Our most recent review suggested that you might benefit from taking low-dose (81mg) aspirin once a day to reduce your risk of having a heart attack or stroke. That may or may not be correct, or you may already be taking low-dose aspirin and we simply haven't recorded it in your record. Low-dose aspirin should only be taken by adults who are at increased risk for a heart attack or stroke, are not allergic to aspirin, and do not have a history of bleeding problems. We suggest that you take the following steps:

If you are no longer a patient of our practice, please call and let us know so that we can remove your record from our active file.

If you are taking low-dose aspirin daily, please contact our office and let us know so that we can put it in your record.

If you are allergic to aspirin or are at increased risk for serious bleeding (e.g. aneurysm, bleeding disorder), please contact our office to make sure we have that information and that it will be considered in future quality reviews.

If you do not believe that you are at increased risk for having a heart attack or stroke, make a note to discuss that with your doctor at your next appointment.

If you believe that you are at increased risk for having a heart attack or stroke, and you are not taking low-dose aspirin, please consider either calling us for advice or making an appointment to discuss it with your doctor.

Thank you for your attention to this important matter, and thank you for trusting us for your primary health care.

Sincerely,
Dr. Paul Jones

As is probably obvious, the chances are good that such a letter was generated automatically by a computer program linked to your doctor's electronic medical record.

In an effort to help doctors move from predominantly acute care (infections and accidents, etc.) to chronic, longitudinal care (diabetes, chronic lung disease, etc.), researchers at the McColl Institute in Seattle and the University of California at San Francisco developed a conceptual approach called "The Care Model," which has served as a map for improving the delivery of primary care. One component of the model involves the use of "registries" to manage populations of patients – as compared to the one-patient-at-a-time approach.

A registry electronically receives and stores information on all patients in a doctor's practice with a particular health condition (e.g., diabetes) from which various analyses and reports can be produced. That makes it possible to contact

patients who have not met their guideline-based targets, and
it helps the practice meet the guideline-based quality metrics
upon which they are increasingly judged and reimbursed.

In the advanced primary care practice envisioned by many
experts and already implemented in a number of health
systems, information collected during ordinary medical care
electronically populates computerized registries. The registries periodically produce lists of patients who, for whatever
reasons, have not had all of the recommended visits, tests,
or procedures the guidelines suggest they should have had.
Those patients are then contacted, either by computer-gen-
erated letter, e-mail, or phone, and advised to come in to
remedy the situation. Flags also appear in the electronic
medical record reminding physicians to take care of the
deficiencies during visits scheduled for other reasons.

Nearly all current registries are disease-based, with a separate
registry for each disease for which guidelines exist.

In concept, registries make a great deal of sense. Their purpose is to systematize care so that important clinical strategies are not forgotten. However, disease-specific registries
reinforce problem-oriented behavior in at least three ways:
1) by focusing on disease-oriented strategies and metrics
rather than meaningful outcomes (goals); 2) by shifting
decision-making from doctors to office staff or to automated
notification systems; and 3) by creating subtle pressure to
clean up the task list even when some tasks wouldn't otherwise be considered necessary.

A Goal-Directed Registry

Registries do not have to be disease-oriented. Over the last 25 years, I have been involved in the development of a goal-directed registry focused primarily on prevention of premature death and disability. For each individual, the registry's computer program considers up to 215 different risk factors, then calculates current life expectancy (ELE) and health expectancy (EHE). It then calculates a "real age," a wellness score," and a quality of life and health score, and it summarizes both strengths and challenges. It then produces a list of preventive measures worth considering. For each preventive measure it shows the size of its expected benefit on life expectancy. Here's what a typical report looks like.

(45 years old - ELE: 81.1 - EHE: 74.6) ❓

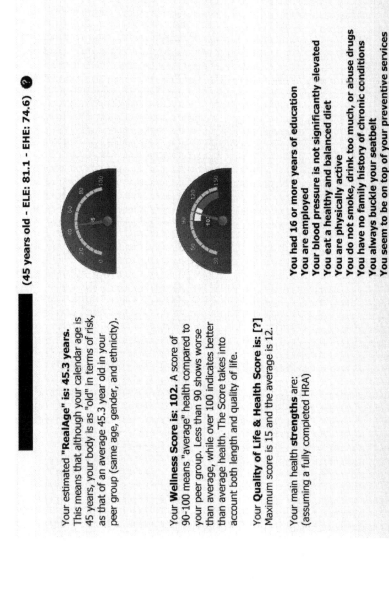

Your estimated **"RealAge" is: 45.3 years.**
This means that although your calendar age is 45 years, your body is as "old" in terms of risk, as that of an average 45.3 year old in your peer group (same age, gender, and ethnicity).

Your **Wellness Score is: 102.** A score of 90-100 means "average" health compared to your peer group. Less than 90 shows worse than average, while over 100 indicates better than average health. The Score takes into account both length and quality of life.

Your **Quality of Life & Health Score is: [?]**
Maximum score is 15 and the average is 12.

Your main health **strengths** are:
(assuming a fully completed HRA)

You had 16 or more years of education
You are employed
Your blood pressure is not significantly elevated
You eat a healthy and balanced diet
You are physically active
You do not smoke, drink too much, or abuse drugs
You have no family history of chronic conditions
You always buckle your seatbelt
You seem to be on top of your preventive services

Your main health **challenges** are:
(assuming a fully completed HRA)

Your life is stressful
You may need to address the amount of sleep you get
Your exposure to unhealthy materials is elevated
Your risk of injury from a car accident is elevated
You do not always wear a helmet when you should
Your risk of sexually transmitted disease may be elevated
You may need to address the management of life challenges

Maximum **health benefit** that can be gained
when all services are completed or maintained:

6.91 additional years of life

Preventive services **ranked** in a decreasing
order of health benefit:

Preventive Services		Share of Benefit
Stress reduction	<--	Link to Resources
Weight control	<--	Link to Resources
Adjusting sleeping time	<--	Link to Resources
Cholesterol measurement	<--	Link to Resources
PAP smear	<--	Link to Resources
Mammography	<--	Link to Resources
Seatbelt use	<--	Link to Resources
Sun exposure protection	<--	Link to Resources
Adult dT-Tdap	<--	Link to Resources
Folic acid supplementation	<--	Link to Resources
Pneumonia vaccination	<--	Link to Resources

While this particular registry has been offered as a stand-alone service by health systems and insurance companies, it is probably more effective when used to inform discussions between individuals and their primary care physicians. Preliminary studies involving use of the registry have found that people who received the registry report and discussed it with their doctor received more high impact preventive services and increased their estimated life expectancy more than those who simply completed the risk factor questionnaire but did not receive the report.

CHAPTER 10:
A Different Kind of Knowledge

"I did then what I knew how to do. Now that I know better, I do better."

—*Maya Angelou*

"Your assumptions are your windows on the world. Scrub them off every once in a while, or the light won't come in."

—*Isaac Asimov*

The way we look at things influences the questions we ask and the methods we use to answer them. Since medical research has primarily focused on questions related to problem solving, research methods have been designed for that purpose, and so that is what we know the most about. In other words, we know a lot about what *can* be done to correct abnormalities, but we know much less about what *should* be done to help people achieve their health goals. Granted there is a fair amount of overlap, but the gaps are still quite significant.

Before we discuss issues involving research questions and methods, it is important to understand a little bit about how problem-oriented research has affected clinical care.

Disease Definitions

To guide research about diseases, disease definitions have been developed. These definitions, which are also called diagnostic criteria, are usually developed by subspecialty experts. An example of this is the Diagnostic and Statistical Manual (DSM) of Mental Disorders, developed by a panel of psychiatrists and psychologists. Here is their definition for a "major depressive episode" from the Fourth Edition of the DSM.

Major Depressive Episode

1. At least five of the following symptoms have been present during the same two-week period, nearly every day, and represent a change from previous functioning. At least one of the symptoms must be either (1) depressed mood or (2) loss of interest or pleasure:

   a. Depressed mood (or irritable mood in children or adolescents)

   b. Markedly diminished interest or pleasure in all, or almost all, activities

   c. Significant weight loss or weight gain when not dieting

    d. Insomnia or hypersomnia

    e. Psychomotor agitation or retardation

    f. Fatigue or loss of energy

    g. Feelings of worthlessness or excessive or inappropriate guilt

    h. Diminished ability to think or concentrate

    i. Recurrent thoughts of death, recurrent suicidal ideation without a specific plan, or a suicide attempt or a specific plan for committing suicide

2. Symptoms are not better accounted for by a Mood Disorder Due to a General Medical Condition, a Substance-Induced Mood Disorder, or Bereavement (normal reaction to the death of a loved one).

3. Symptoms are not better accounted for by a Psychotic Disorder (e.g. Schizoaffective Disorder).

While the DSM was created for research purposes, it has been widely adopted by physicians for management of patients. In fact, the quality of care provided by physicians is often judged based upon whether the diagnostic criteria have been documented and whether treatments prescribed are justified by diagnoses. That all sounds reasonable unless you have actually suffered from depression or have tried to help someone who is depressed.

Depression is far too common in our society. Many people meet the criteria for major depressive episode at some time in their lives – and each of them is unique. Their circumstances, personal resources, family and social support, vulnerabilities, and (yes) goals are different. And while they might share some common biological abnormalities, the factors contributing to their symptoms are as different as they are.

However, the process of putting a name and definition around a set of symptoms tends to shift the focus toward the condition and away from the person who has the symptoms. It gives physicians the sense, once they have determined that the person meets the definition of major depressive episode, that they understand what is going on. Influenced by time and energy constraints and supported by guidelines and the pharmaceutical companies, they learn to link diagnoses to drugs. When I say, "depression" – physicians think, "SSRI" (a type of antidepressant).

Goal-directed care would require that the focus of research be on goal-attainment, not problem-solving. When problem-solving contributes to goal-attainment, there is overlap, so knowledge gained from disease-based research is still useful. However, a shift to goal-directed care would require a corresponding shift in the focus and design of research studies in order to fill the gaps that would become apparent.

Prevention of Premature Death and Disability

Goal attainment differs from problem solving in several ways. In the case of life extension, the timeline is much longer. The greatest challenge for researchers studying life extension is that risk factors often take years to have their effects, and it has been hard for researchers to get funding to conduct studies lasting longer than 3 - 5 years. As a result, the actual benefits of many preventive measures can only be estimated.

Because autopsies are rarely performed anymore, the best available information on causes of death in the general population still comes from death certificates, which, according to a 2010 survey of the doctors in New York City responsible for completing them, are often inaccurate. Supporting that view, a study conducted in 2012 in England found that the reported cause of death was inaccurate 22% of the time and grossly inaccurate 20% of the time when compared to autopsy findings.

Most of the information we have about the impact of health care on survival, therefore, pertains only to people with a single disease that is likely to cause death in the very near future (e.g., severe heart disease). And for most diseases, we don't really know whether treatment improves survival or by how much and at what cost.

Try asking your doctor how much longer, on average, you are likely to live if you control your blood sugar levels better or take your heart medicines or lose 20 pounds. Then try to find the answers to those questions on the Internet. How can you be expected to make truly informed decisions about which life extension strategies to choose when the information you need to make those decisions is not available?

Implementation of a goal-directed approach would require more information from a broader range of people followed over longer periods of time. This could be done prospectively (people followed into the future) or retrospectively (people followed in the past, for instance by life insurance companies), perhaps complemented by computer modeling techniques based upon our increasingly sophisticated understanding of human biology. From such information it should be possible to create and improve predictive algorithms like the one described earlier.

Goals also involve trade-offs. In order to decide whether treatment of a disease is a good idea, you must not only consider whether the treatment could extend your life but whether the extra life it could provide would be worth the effort. For example, if sleeping an extra hour each night increased your life expectancy by 5 months over a ten year period, it would be important to know if all or most of that additional time would be spent sleeping.

Quality of Life

It should now be clear to you, if it wasn't already, that quality of life means very different things to different people. That creates at least two challenges for researchers, both of which have solutions.

The first challenge is how to measure the success of a treatment intended to improve quality of life. The standard approach is to measure relief of symptoms, improvement in standard functions like walking speed, physical signs, and test results – the same measures for every person in the experiment. However, there is no particular reason why the outcome of interest couldn't be different for each person as long as the measures of interest were defined prior to the experiment. For example, the outcome could be whether or not participants improved their ability to participate in the activities each considered important.

The second challenge is that the strategies for improving quality of life are also likely to different for each individual. This challenge could be met by studying evaluation and decision-making *processes* rather than predetermined strategies. For example, rather than studying whether a specific medicine or surgical procedure improves the abilities of participants to achieve their quality of life goals, researchers could instead study whether having an evaluation by an occupational therapist followed by development of a treatment plan is more effective than the standard medical approach. When this sort of experiment has been done, by the way, occupational therapy has nearly always been shown to be more effective than standard care.

I have mentioned occupational therapists several times now. Occupational therapists are health care professionals whose job is to help people do the things they want and need to do. Naturally, a majority of them work in rehabilitation settings helping people with disabilities, but many work in schools, workplaces, nursing homes, and people's homes (See _www.aota.org_). Medicare, Medicaid, and most insurance companies require a physician referral before they will pay for occupational therapy services.

A Good Death

Though recommendations abound, surprisingly little research has been done to determine the best ways to prepare for a good death. As with quality of life, values and preferences for care at the end of life differ significantly between different individuals. So, just as for quality of life, outcomes should be individualized and studies should evaluate processes that could result in individualized strategies for achieving a good death as defined by each person.

Personal Growth and Development

Growth and development have typically been studied by psychologists who have focused primarily on children. However, aside from the attention paid to developmental milestones during well-child care visits, that knowledge has had little impact on health care. A goal-directed approach would require better measures of personal growth and development and more studies examining the impact of various health care interventions on them.

An area of research leading the way in this regard involves "health literacy." Health literacy is defined as the degree to which individuals have the capacity to obtain, process, and understand basic health information and services needed to make appropriate health decisions (*https://health.gov*). Much has already been learned about how the health care system can both assess and improve health literacy, a critical component of successful growth and development.

As mentioned in an earlier chapter, other health-related developmental areas needing further study include 1) mastery of the skills required for healthy living; 2) increasing the motivation to maintain and improve health; 3) integration within a social network and the relational skills necessary to do that; and 4) the habits of self-assessment, reflection, goal-setting, and self-directed learning.

Decision-making Processes

To fully implement goal-directed health care we would also need to know more about goal-setting and strategic planning. Fortunately, other fields (e.g., education, mental health, financial planning, business, etc.) have lots of experience using a goal-directed approach, and much of that knowledge should be applicable. However, some challenges would probably be unique to health care.

What You Can Do

I'm sure many of you are wondering why I included a chapter on research in a book intended for a lay audience. As with all of the chapters in this section, my primary purpose was to help you understand what you are up against and why. In this case, if you ask the right questions, you will often discover that the answers are not available, because they haven't been asked before or because answering them would be difficult using current methods. All you can do is to explain why the questions are important, and support researchers willing to try to answer them.

There are actually at least three ways you can support goal-directed research: 1) volunteer to participate as a research subject; 2) join a patient advisory group connected to a research institution or funding agency so that you can help shape the research agenda; and 3) encourage Congress and other research funders to support research that attempts to answer the questions important to people like you.

There are several ways to find out about opportunities to participate in goal-relevant research. If you live somewhere near a university health center, call their Office of Research Administration, and ask for information about "clinical research" being conducted on campus and how to get involved. Only sign up for studies designed to answer questions you find relevant and important. Research conducted by faculty in Occupational Therapy, Family Medicine, General Internal Medicine, Pediatrics, Sports Medicine, or Geriatrics is most likely to address the kinds of issues discussed in this book.

CHAPTER 11:

Goal-Directed Care and Health Care Reform

Over the past three decades policy makers have made a concerted effort to reform health care, primarily because it costs so much. Recent strategies have focused on the "Triple Aim," a concept developed by Donald Berwick, former Director of the Centers for Medicare and Medicaid Services, which includes: (1) improving the quality of the care provided, (2) improving patient outcomes including satisfaction with care, and (3) reducing cost. As you will see, a goal-directed approach could improve all three.

Quality of Health Care

Whether goal-directed care would improve the quality of health care would depend upon how quality was defined and measured. Currently, quality of care is judged based upon the degree to which health care providers have followed disease-oriented guidelines, and the degree to which their patients have achieved recommended levels of disease control.

For example, quality of care for patients with diabetes is graded based upon whether certain examinations (eye and foot examinations) or tests (average blood sugar and cholesterol) were performed and the percentage of patients with average blood sugar levels above 212 (A1c of 9) and below 183 (A1c of 8).

Many primary care doctors complain about these quality measures for two very good reasons. First, they are based on the assumption that all patients with the same condition should receive the same treatment – cookbook medicine. Second, doctors object to being judged on quality measures that require substantial cooperation on the part of their patients. In other words, they feel they are being penalized when patients don't follow their advice. As insurance payments to physicians become more tightly linked to this kind of quality measurement, there is concern that some doctors will refuse to see patients who they believe to be less able or willing to follow recommendations.

In sharp contrast to this problem-oriented view of quality, G. E. Steffen, frustrated by years of work as a quality improvement professional, wrote the following in an article published in 1988 in the *Journal of the American Medical Association*, "For the physician and patient, quality of medical care can be defined as that care that has the capacity to achieve the goals of the physician and the patient." He also pointed out that, in most cases, the goals of health care actions are not documented in the medical record, making accurate quality assessment impossible.

So, whether a goal-directed approach would improve the quality of health care would depend upon which definition of "quality" one chose to use. The problem-oriented approach assumes that everyone with the same health conditions should receive approximately the same treatment. The goal-directed approach assumes that every person is unique, and that high-quality health care should assure that each person is treated differently based upon their personal goals, challenges, resources, values, and preferences.

For example, many people will benefit very little or not at all from blood pressure reduction including those with a limited life expectancy, those for whom life prolongation is no longer a goal, those who will certainly die from something other than a stroke or heart attack because of other health challenges (e.g., alcoholism), and those who are unable or unwilling to do what it would take to lower their blood pressure. Goal-directed care would assure that each patient's unique situation and individual goals would be taken into account when deciding whether or not to prescribe blood pressure medications.

If quality was defined as care that is likely to help each patient achieve better health as they define it, then goal-directed care would be of higher quality than problem-oriented care for several reasons. First, because goal-directed care focuses directly on achievement of patient goals rather than indirectly through problem-solving, the strategies chosen would be more likely to be relevant and feasible. And, as illustrated by the cases discussed earlier, the range of strategies would be wider since they would not be limited to problem-solving.

Returning to the example of the man with severe chronic obstructive lung disease who required oxygen therapy, instruction in hand washing, regular dental care, and avoidance of contact with people with viral illnesses would, in a goal-directed approach, characterize higher quality care than excellent cholesterol and blood pressure management, even though those measures might be justifiable based upon disease-based guidelines.

In addition, when doctors and patients develop plans collaboratively based upon agreed upon goals, patients are more likely to adhere to them… more likely to keep follow-up appointments, fill and take their medicines, and live in healthy ways, etc. Therefore, rather than being a concern, the degree to which a plan was followed could be a reasonable gauge of the quality of the care that was provided. In this case, however, "adherence" would be adherence to an individualized plan rather than to a plan based upon a disease-specific guideline.

Disparities in the quality of care received based upon age, gender, race, income, insurance, education, transportation, and disabilities are a major challenge for our health care system and the health of the country. Some people receive excellent care while others receive either very poor or no health care at all. At least some of these disparities are rooted in deep-seated societal prejudices and cultural misunderstandings. A goal-directed approach could help reduce some of these disparities. Prejudices are strongest when the individuals involved don't know each other. Because goal-directed care depends upon understanding each person as a unique human being, prejudices might be reduced.

In the university teaching clinics where I taught, a majority of the patients were economically and socially disadvantaged. When supervising the physicians-in-training, I watched their attitudes toward patients progress from hopelessness and frustration – because they could see no way to make their patients "normal" - to compassion, empathy, admiration, and collaboration as they got to know them better over time. That led to a higher level of investment on the part of both physicians and patients in improved health outcomes.

Physicians who live and work in the same community for long periods of time tend to become goal-directed as their relationships with their patients and their investment in their well-being increase over time. A goal-directed approach could hasten and strengthen this process since getting to know patients is essential to the model rather than something that might or might not occur over time as a byproduct of problem-solving.

Health Care Outcomes

The benefits of health care to patients should also be greater as a result of a goal-directed approach, because the outcomes that mattered to each person would be the direct focus of the care provided. And because the strategies devised to achieve those outcomes would be personalized, they would be easier for patients to implement. Yogi Berra once said, "If you don't know where you are going, you'll end up someplace else." Unfortunately that happens in our current health care system all the time.

Very early in my medical career I took care of a woman who I will call Betty. Betty had Type 2 (adult onset) diabetes, which should have been easy to control with diet and a couple of medications. Although she checked her blood sugars at home every day, Betty insisted that she also have her blood sugars checked in the office once a week. To my increasing dismay, despite my best efforts, her blood sugar levels both at home and in the office were always high – in the mid 200s, twice as high as I would have liked.

Confused and frustrated, I admitted Betty to the hospital for further testing and to see if her blood sugar elevation might be because she wasn't following my advice. Sure enough, her blood sugar levels came right down to normal in the hospital on the medications she had been told to take and the diet she was told to follow. After reviewing her condition and its treatment with her again, I discharged her and told her, as nicely as I could, that there was no point in coming to the office every week until she was willing and able to take her medicines and to stick to her diet.

And she fired me.

I later learned through the grapevine that visiting the clinic every week was a major social activity for Betty, and I theorized that she believed that allowing her blood sugars to remain high would justify the weekly visits. If this was indeed the case, then her quality of life goal would have been in direct conflict with my disease management goal. I'd like to think that later in my career I would have recognized this, and we could have developed a plan to satisfy Betty's socialization need while allowing her to benefit from better blood sugar control.

Patient satisfaction with care is another way to measure outcomes. A goal-directed approach should increase patient satisfaction in several obvious ways. First, the values, knowledge and opinions that each patient brings to the doctor-patient relationship would be valued. This would not only improve the quality of the relationship, but it would support patient self-confidence and physician empathy, requirements for emotional well-being.

The Cost of Health Care

Goal-directed care would also be less expensive than problem-oriented care. First, as we have seen, there would almost certainly be fewer tests and treatments because of the direct focus on meaningful outcomes – outcomes that matter to patients. By choosing diagnostic and therapeutic strategies with the greatest potential impact for each person, benefits would be maximized and costs reduced. And because the focus of the doctor-patient relationship would be on goal achievement rather than disease management, the range of strategies would be greater, including more low-cost options like hand washing, avoiding sick children, and dental hygiene.

Second, because of a lifespan view of health and the personal growth and development goal, greater value would be placed on giving natural healing processes an opportunity to work. The focus of care would shift from what *could* be done to what *should* be done. That would mean, for example, fewer antibiotics. And because of the "good death" goal, advance directives would be completed by more people, preventing many unwanted interventions at the end of life.

As discussed earlier, curing or managing diseases does not necessarily result in restoration of function. Because of the direct focus on improving and maintaining the ability to function, indirect economic benefits could include increased productivity of patients at work, school, and home.

Finally, closer relationships between doctors and their patients should reduce the number of malpractice suits, lowering insurance premiums over time and reducing unnecessary tests and treatments done simply to prevent successful lawsuits.

In summary, a goal-oriented definition of health and a goal-directed approach to health care could be expected to improve quality of care and patient outcomes while at the same time reducing costs. It would therefore be a great way to achieve the Triple Aims.

SECTION 3:
Achieving your Health Goals

"Eat good food, not too much, mostly vegetables."

—Michael Pollan in The Omnivore's Dilemma

"Get good health care, not too much, mostly primary care."

—Kevin Grumbach,
Chairman of Family Medicine at UCSF

In this section I will discuss how to avoid getting too much health care, the importance of getting mostly primary care, and finally how to get good health care. My purpose is to help you to achieve your personal health goals, and, when necessary, wrestle goal-directed care out of the problem-oriented health care system. I hope that in doing so, you will also have a positive influence on the health care system.

CHAPTER 12:

Limiting Your Exposure to the Health Care System

"For many years, both doctors and patients have had a 'more is better' attitude. It is time to adopt a 'think twice' attitude and to avoid unnecessary and potentially harmful tests, procedures and treatment."

—*Wendy Levinson*

"Often the best medicine is no medicine at all, or the best intervention is no intervention at all. But those conversations with patients that take time to explain that the evidence simply doesn't support doing a test or prescribing a drug are long conversations, and it's much easier in clinical practice to do things quickly and prescribe or order a test."

—*Rachelle Buchbinder*

Nearly everyone can benefit from health care at some point during his or her life. You may need the health care system to help you face life threatening challenges. You might need the knowledge of health care professionals when the causes of your symptoms are unclear. And you will probably benefit from immunizations and screening tests, as well as from advice and assistance when health-related obstacles prevent you from enjoying activities important to your quality of life.

However, while the health care system can both extend and improve the quality of your life, it can also cause great harm. Medical errors are now the third leading cause of death in the United States. More than 100,000 people each year die from the adverse effects of medicines that were prescribed *correctly*. In an attempt to eliminate disease and discomfort, the health care system has a tendency to over-test, over-diagnose, and over-treat, causing physical, psychological, and financial harm to many people.

For that reason it is important that you obtain health care only when necessary.

The best way to avoid getting too much health care is to focus on your goals.

Remember, our health care system is really good at fixing things. And you will almost certainly need to have some things fixed from time to time. But, as we've seen, the current problem-oriented system isn't very good at figuring out *which* things need to be fixed and *when* it is necessary to step in and try to fix them. That is where you will have to come in.

Take Care of Yourself

The best way to limit your number of contacts with the health care system is to stay healthy and to reduce your risk of premature death and disability by taking certain precautions. Consider how well you would take care of your car if you knew it had to last for 90 to 100 years. You would probably change the oil and filters regularly, apply wax and other sun damage protectants, take it in for regular maintenance, and develop an ongoing relationship with a mechanic. You might even drive more carefully. A popular greeting card reads, "If I'd known I was going to live this long I'd have taken better care of myself." Heed that warning!

For survival, human beings need food, water, sleep, and physical activity. Good health requires getting enough but not too much of each of those things. Though we are still learning a great deal about nutrition, it is clear that we need a mixture of food types – particularly fruits and vegetables – in quantities sufficient to maintain a body mass index (weight divided by height squared) of between 22 and 26. We probably need to drink about 2 ½ quarts of liquid a day, more when it's hot, when we have a fever, and when we are exercising vigorously. Most people seem to need between six and nine hours of sleep per night and at least 2 ½ hours of moderate physical activity per week. Moderate physical activity is activity that is strenuous enough so that you can still talk but not sing, maintained for at least 10 minutes at a time. If you need some motivation to become more physically active, I recommend that you read *Younger Next Year* by Crowley and Lodge. Be aware that the book has two versions, one for men and another for women, so get the right version for you.

Studies have shown that you are likely to live longer if you continue your formal education beyond high school and your informal education throughout your life. In addition to affecting the kinds of jobs that will be available to you and your level of income, the things you learn will prepare you to make better decisions about your health and health care.

You are also less likely to become ill or die prematurely if you: live in a safe environment; either don't own guns or practice safe gun ownership; wear a helmet when riding a bike or motorcycle; wear a life jacket when riding in a boat; and learn ways to handle emotional stress.

Smoking cigarettes is one of the best ways to shorten your life and to make death a miserable experience. Each cigarette you smoke shortens your life by an average of 11 minutes. Smoking increases the risk for almost every known disease. If your goal is to live as long as possible and avoid doctors and hospitals, don't smoke! Cigar, pipe, and chewing tobacco use may be less hazardous to your lungs, but those forms of tobacco still increase your risk for mouth, throat, and esophageal cancers as well as other diseases.

We all want to believe that we have complete control over our thoughts and actions. We believe, for example, that we won't become addicted to anything. While it is true that some people are more susceptible to addiction than others, no one is immune. If family members have had problems with addiction, you should be particularly cautious. Addictive substances (alcohol, tobacco, opiates, anti-anxiety medications, marijuana, amphetamines, etc.) and behaviors (e.g., gambling, shopping, eating, pornography, etc.) can change your brain chemistry and pathways, taking away the control that you thought you would always have. Be very careful! Those brain changes are extremely hard, sometimes impossible, to reverse.

Prevent Preventable Illnesses

Immunizations are easy, inexpensive, and extremely safe. In many cases, they not only protect you or your children directly, but, by increasing the level of resistance in the population, some immunizations can also protect you indirectly through "herd immunity." However, we currently only have immunizations for a few potentially serious infections.

Other infections can be avoided by knowing how they are spread. Most common infections are caused by viruses. Viruses often spread through the air or in food. If possible, stay away from people with viral infections (e.g., coughs, congestion, diarrhea, etc.), and try hard not to expose others to your illnesses. When exposure is unknown or unavoidable, wash your hands after potential exposures, for example before touching your eyes or nose since viruses are often acquired from contaminated surfaces.

Depending upon your particular risk factors, it might make sense to take certain medicines (e.g., aspirin or cholesterol medicine) or have certain procedures (e.g., mastectomy) to prevent the development of serious health challenges to which you are susceptible. Those decisions will obviously require consultation with your doctors.

As discussed earlier, screening tests (e.g. pap smears, mammograms, colonoscopies, hepatitis C blood tests, etc.) are tests used to detect major health challenges before they cause symptoms. It makes sense to have certain screening tests done, but only if you plan to act on the results. For example, don't agree to have a prostate specific antigen blood test unless you plan to have biopsies followed by treatment with either surgery or radiation if the test is positive. And, of course, when staying alive is no longer a goal for you, don't agree to be screened for anything.

Careful management of chronic (ongoing) health challenges can increase survival, improve quality of life, or both. But before agreeing to treatment for any chronic health condition, try to find out whether and how much the treatment is likely to impact your goals. You may find that a particular treatment may not be relevant to you. Again, many people have had a coronary artery bypass operation to improve circulation to the heart muscle, thinking that it will prolong their lives. In fact, the main benefit of this commonly performed operation is relief of chest pain. If you don't have chest pain, with only few exceptions, you probably won't benefit. However, many cardiologists and cardiac surgeons have a hard time resisting the urge to open up clogged arteries, restoring normal blood flow, and they have a significant financial incentive to do so.

Understand and Address your Vulnerabilities

Each of us has a unique set of vulnerabilities, which put us at increased risk for specific health challenges. Some vulnerabilities are inherited and some result from events and circumstances.

Because so much about us is determined by our genes, it is important to find out as much as possible about the vulnerabilities and health challenges experienced by members of your biological family. How old were they when they died? What caused their deaths? What caused them to become disabled if they did? Which medicines did they do well on, and which ones caused problems for them or didn't work. Draw a genogram (*http://stanfield.pbworks.com/f/explaining_genograms.pdf*), and include health-related information. Once you have identified the types of health challenges that run in your family, learn everything you can about them and particularly how to prevent them.

Risk calculators are now available to help you determine your vulnerability to a variety of common health challenges. Since most people in the United States die of a heart attack or stroke, you may want to use one of the online cardiovascular risk calculators like the ones at *http://tools.acc.org/ASCVD-Risk-Estimator*, *http://cvdrisk.nhlbi.nih.gov*, or *http://www.reynoldsriskscore.org* to determine your risk for a heart attack or stroke. You can calculate your risk for a variety of cancers at *http://www.yourdiseaserisk.wustl.edu/YDRDefault.aspx?ScreenControl=YDRGeneral&ScreenName=YDRCancer_Index*.

Remember your Goals

You will find that when you are clear with yourself and your doctors about the things that matter most to you, you will be more likely to get what you need from the health care system in fewer visits. Conversely, when your goals are unclear, you are more likely to end up, like Brer Rabbit in the Uncle Remus stories, "stuck in the tar" – in this case the sticky tentacles of the health care system.

Think about a typical day in your life and the things that you need and want to be able to do. Then think about your passions, the activities without which life would no longer be meaningful or enjoyable. As you think about these things, remember that eliminating a problem (e.g., curing a disease) is not the same as achieving a goal, though it might be an important strategy or objective.

A friend of mine has had psoriasis for most of his adult life. When he was employed as a sales manager for an information technology company, he had to meet with lots of people every day. One of his goals was to have a successful and fulfilling career and provide for his family. At that time, his psoriasis presented a challenge. He was embarrassed by the rash, which required that he wear long sleeve shirts, and the lesions often bled through his shirt sleeves. After trying a variety of creams and ointments, he saw a dermatologist who treated him with a powerful medication, which controlled the psoriasis but also damaged the nerves in his feet causing permanent numbness and some discomfort. He did enjoy a very successful career, and so, probably, the downside was worth it.

Now he is retired and can manage his rash well enough with creams and ointments to do the things he wants and needs to do (e.g., write, travel, and entertain friends). He has considered trying a different oral or injectable medicine to better control his condition, but he has concluded that, while it might improve his appearance, it wouldn't really make his quality of life any better. At this point the risk of adverse medication effects isn't worth the benefits.

Achieving your goals often requires combinations of strategies. Let's say your goal is to be able to go on walks with your grandchildren. You may need to do exercises to improve strength, flexibility, or balance. There may be specific treatments that would be helpful (e.g., joint replacement). Better management of specific medical problems (e.g., diabetes, anemia, heart failure, etc.) could also help. If the physical obstacles can't be overcome, you may need to find ways around them, like using a cane, a walker, or even a scooter or electric wheelchair.

Use Medicines Cautiously

Very few medicines actually prolong life. Notable exceptions include antibiotics for life threatening infections, medicines like aspirin and statins that can reduce the risk of a fatal heart attack or stroke, several medicines that slow the progression of heart failure, and some medicines used to treat cancer. The primary purpose of most medicines is to relieve symptoms. Most symptoms have a purpose, and all medicines can cause side effects, but, out of a desire to do something to make you feel better, *both you and your doctor will nearly always overestimate the benefits and underestimate the hazards of medications.*

Whether you believe, as I do, that the way our bodies work is the result of hundreds of millions of years of natural selection or the result of intelligent design, when you develop a symptom, your first assumption should be that the symptom has a valid purpose. Sneezing and coughing help to clear germs from your nose and lungs. Diarrhea helps to clear germs and other harmful materials from your bowels. Fever also seems to help your body get rid of germs. Inflammation, while painful serves an important role in healing damaged muscles and joints. When you take medicines to block these symptoms, you are essentially saying that you know more than Mother Nature (or God) about how your body should handle the situation. Having said that, sometimes the benefit of the symptom is probably outweighed by the distress it causes, and sometimes the body seems to over-react to threats. I suggest erring on the side of non-interference unless the symptoms are interfering with really important functions like sleeping and eating.

It can be difficult to figure out whether a medicine is actually helping and whether you are experiencing side effects. For that reason, when the purpose of a medicine is long-term symptom relief, keep a diary of *all* of your symptoms for 2 weeks before and 2 weeks after starting the medicine. You will then have a better idea about how much it actually helps and whether it is causing trouble. Also, consider stopping symptom-relief medicines – one at a time, every so often – to see if you still need them. Give your body a couple of weeks to readjust before deciding whether or not to restart a medicine. Sometimes it even makes sense to take symptom-relief medicines just 3 weeks per month, giving your body one week each month to recover and readjust.

Whenever you develop a new symptom, if you are already taking one or more medicines, the first question you should ask yourself is, "Could this be a side effect of one of my medicines?" Unless you and your doctor consider that possibility first, you could easily end up having unnecessary tests and treatments when the solution is to stop a medicine. Because side effects are difficult to recognize, doctors often unwittingly prescribe additional medicines to treat the side effects of previous medicines. For example, patients taking arthritis medicines often develop fluid retention or elevated blood pressure, which prompts their doctors to prescribe diuretics. The diuretics can result in losses of potassium and magnesium leading to prescriptions for supplements.

Most medicines are designed to target individual chemical reactions in the body. For example, antihistamines attach to histamine receptors on cells, preventing the histamine produced by your body in response to allergens from causing its usual effects, nasal congestion and sneezing. But our bodies are incredibly complex. When one process is altered by a medicine, others are always affected as well. For example, antihistamines inhibit saliva production, which can alter the balance of germs in the mouth, increasing the risk of cavities and gingivitis. They also reduce muscle contractions in the bowel causing some people to be constipated.

Medication side effects are often subtle or confusing. Someone taking a medicine for osteoporosis may not recognize that their low back pain is not due to the osteoporosis but is a side effect of the medicine they are taking to treat it. A person taking a medicine to block stomach acid may not realize that it is the reason they have been having more headaches. Anxiety, depression, and fatigue are all side effects of a number of commonly used medicines. They often develop gradually and are mistakenly attributed to life events.

Medicines also interact with each other, with foods, and with chronic health conditions. Simple interactions between medicines can be predicted and avoided by using widely available computer programs available to all pharmacists and most doctors. However, it is practically impossible to predict interactions between three or more medicines. And beyond about five medicines, the benefits of the individual medications are usually outweighed by their unwanted side effects and interactions.

So, in order to reduce your contacts with the health care system, limit the number of medicines you take, and, if multiple medicines are required, try to keep the total number below 5. I hope that sounds to most of you like a lot of medicines. It is. Shockingly, 30% of people over 65 take 8 or more prescription medicines daily. My personal record was a patient who was taking 27 different medicines every day when I first met her.

Medicines, when used properly and in moderation, can make life more pleasant and can occasionally be lifesaving.

For those reasons they are the source of incredible profits for pharmaceutical companies, which now spend close to $5 billion per year on direct-to-you commercials and advertisements—the consumer-ads for new medications. More than 80 of these ads are now shown per hour on television in the U.S.

My advice to you: Mute the TV or leave the room during pharmaceutical commercials. If you are unable to take your eyes off of the TV screen, see if you can figure out how the pharmaceutical companies come up with the names they are giving to new drugs. It looks like they pick letters at random from a Scrabble set that has been enriched with v's, x's, and z's.

There are at least four reasons to ignore pharmaceutical company advertisements:

1. The medicine being pushed is probably no more effective than older alternatives. When a new medicine is a breakthrough, it is the subject of news reports and announcements to physicians. Everyone will know about it already.

2. All of the ads promote newer, brand name medications, not generics. They are therefore guaranteed to be much more expensive than prior medications used for the same conditions.

3. The ads, by design, paint the rosiest possible picture of the new medicine. Side effects are always downplayed in a variety of subtle and not so subtle ways.

4. The ads are effective. The pharmaceutical industry has estimated a 5:1 return on investment for direct-to-consumer advertisements. If you pay attention to the ads, you are likely to end up on more medications, which will almost certainly mean more encounters with the health care system.

Several excellent books have been written about the promotion and overuse of medicines. These include *Overtreated* by Shannon Brownlee, *Overdosed America* by John Abramson, and *How We Do Harm* by Otis Webb Brawley. I strongly suggest you read at least one of them.

Discomfort and Disability

Over the last 50 years or so we have come to believe that we shouldn't have to tolerate discomfort. We assume that nearly every health problem can be solved, every abnormality corrected, and every disease cured. Even if that was true, which it isn't of course, fixing every abnormality is not always necessary, or even the right thing to do. A particular patient comes to mind.

Mr. Zeller was a retired attorney who had recently seen a neurosurgeon for back and leg pains. The neurosurgeon told him that he had lumbar spinal stenosis, a condition in which the lower spinal cord is compressed gradually by overgrowth of bone, and that no effective treatment was available. I asked Mr. Zeller about his daily routine and activities. He said that he spent most of his time at the computer writing or in his chair reading. When I asked him how important walking was to him and how bad it would be if he had to get around in a wheelchair, he said, "It wouldn't be that bad." "Then," I said, "don't worry about your spinal stenosis. The worst that could happen, and it may never happen, is that you will lose the ability to walk. It isn't likely to shorten your life." He broke down in tears of gratitude and relief. He thought that when the neurosurgeon had said his condition was incurable, he had sentenced him to a life of discomfort and an early death.

I also remember a conversation I had with my then 14-year-old son. He said, "Dad, it seems like people don't want to have any problems, but I don't think that would necessarily be a good thing." I told him he was wise beyond his years.

In fact, for many of us, facing challenges and overcoming obstacles is rewarding and may actually be essential for optimal physical and psychological development. The way our bodies learn to fight serious infections is by fighting less serious ones. The way we learn to handle big losses is to handle smaller ones.

Become More Self-Sufficient

Avoiding unnecessary contact with the health care system also requires some level of understanding about how your body works. There are many books, newsletters, and Internet websites about health, and you should definitely seek out those kinds of resources. In general, this is a good way to become more self-sufficient.

But, as you know, there is a lot of misinformation out there. Be careful to choose materials written or sanctioned by reputable organizations. Try to avoid information produced or sponsored by the pharmaceutical, nutritional supplement, or medical device industries, or anyone else trying to sell you something. If you have a specific medical condition, consider becoming a member of the national association for that condition.

When you have specific questions between visits to your doctor, the most helpful and accurate source of health information is likely to be a reference librarian at a medical center library. Librarians have been trained to help you find the most current, reliable information on any topic. Make sure that the person helping you knows how you plan to use the information (i.e., your goal).

Of course, the Internet is an easier, more accessible source of information. But beware! Try to stick to sites that don't have a product or service to sell, sites marked "Ad" or whose web address ends in ".com".

I recommend the following sites:
MedlinePlus (*http://www.nlm.nih.gov/medlineplus*)
HealthFinder (*http://www.healthfinder.gov*)
MLA Top Health Websites (*http://www.mlanet.org/consumer*)

Network news reports can sometimes be helpful, but the quality of the information is sometimes misleading. Better sources of information are newsletters produced by reputable academic health centers like the Berkeley Wellness Letter

(*http://www.berkeleywellness.com*) and the Harvard Health
Publications (*http://www.health.harvard.edu*).

I know how hard it can be to decide whether you should see
a doctor when you aren't feeling well. Remember that your
body is incredibly resilient, and it learns from experience.
To paraphrase philosopher Friedrich Nietzsche (and the pop
song by Kelly Clarkson), "What doesn't kill you makes you
stronger." We live in a trigger-happy culture when it comes
to health care, and often, it's smart to put down the gun.

So… aside from the signs and symptoms of a heart attack,
stroke, bleeding aneurysm, or other emergencies, it is usually best to give things a little time to improve on their own
without medical intervention. Remember, when you seek
medical help, the doctor will feel some pressure to do something, even when both of you know it isn't really necessary.

Almost all middle ear, sinus, and bronchial infections get
better just about as quickly without antibiotics, and, when
you allow that to happen, your body develops antibodies,
leaving it better prepared to prevent and handle future
infections. Thus it is usually safe to wait at least 5 days to
see if your body can begin to handle the infection before
asking for help. If you have specific risk factors like a weak
immune system or emphysema, you might need antibiotics
sooner than that. In any case, when you do seek help, make
sure the doctor knows that you only want treatment if it is
absolutely necessary.

Serious health challenges like cancer, which aren't usually emergencies, nearly always get worse over time. Therefore, one of the best ways to figure out whether a new symptom is serious enough to require medical care is to see if it gets better or worse. How long you should wait will depend upon how much the symptoms bother you, but for most symptoms it is generally safe to wait at least a couple of weeks.

Dying Well

Improving the chances of a good death should be a goal for everyone, not just old people. Conflicts and controversies are more likely to occur when young people are critically ill. Don't wait to begin working on this. Fortunately, you and your family can take care of most of the things that can be done ahead of time to increase the likelihood of a good death. The following is a list of actions to consider.

Read *Being Mortal* by Atul Gawande. This well-written, easy-to-read book talks about the interactions that take place between people with life threatening conditions and the health care system, as well as the questions we all should all consider when facing death.

Learn more about advance directives. Places to start include: *https://www.nlm.nih.gov/medlineplus/advancedirectives.html* *https://www.nia.nih.gov/health/publication/end-life-helping-comfort-and-care/planning-end-life-care-decisions*, and *http://www.healthinaging.org/making-your-wishes-known* .

Complete, sign, and make several copies of your state's approved advance directive document or documents. On the internet, search for "advance directive" and the name of your state. Links to these can also be found at: _http://www. caringinfo.org/i4a/pages/index.cfm?pageid=3289_ .

Use the open space provided in these documents to explain conditions you would consider to be worse than death and other issues important to you. Give copies to key family members, friends, and caregivers and be sure they know where you keep them.

Complete and sign a Durable Power of Attorney (DPOA) that includes health care decisions. You can find out more about DPOAs at: _http://www.nolo.com/legal-encyclopedia/ durable-power-of-attorney-health-finances-29579.html_ .

If you can't afford a lawyer or want to do it yourself, a standard form is available at:

https://www.powerofattorney.com/medical-power-attorney/, or your state may provide one.

If you would like to donate your organs to another person when you die, find out how to make that happen in your state. Reliable sources of information include:

http://organdonor.gov/becomingdonor/index.html and _https://www.nlm.nih.gov/medlineplus/organdonation.html._

Think about and discuss with key family members, friends, and caregivers your thoughts and preferences about autopsies, funerals, cremation, and burial arrangements. Make sure someone knows where you keep important documents. The more planning you do, the easier it will be for them.

Ways to Reduce Excessive Exposure to the Health Care System

1. Get enough and the right kinds of food, fluids, physical activity, and sleep.

2. Get as much formal education as possible.

3. Receive high impact (based upon your personal risk profile) preventive care.

4. Avoid addictive substances and behaviors.

5. Always keep your health-related goals clearly in mind when considering an encounter with the health care system.

6. Take medications only when absolutely necessary to achieve your goals.

7. Discuss your health-related goals, values, and preferences with those who might need to participate in decision-making if you are not able to speak for yourself. Complete all available legal forms and give copies to those who might need them.

8. Become a knowledgeable consumer of health care and an expert in the health challenges you currently face or are likely to face in the future by going to reputable sources of information.

CHAPTER 13:
Primary Care

"While the patient wants the best and most modern treatment available, he is also badly in need of the old-fashioned friend that a doctor has always personified…"

—*Gunner Gunderson*

"A person in difficulty wants in the first place the help of another person on whom he can rely as a friend – someone with knowledge of what is feasible but also with good judgment on what is desirable in the particular circumstances and an understanding of what the circumstances are. The more complex medicine becomes, the stronger are the reasons why everyone should have a personal doctor…"

—*T.F. Fox*

As we have discussed, there are now subspecialists (e.g., orthopedists) and even super-subspecialists (e.g., orthopedists who only work on knees) in every conceivable field of medicine and health care more generally. Because of this, one might think that the best approach to getting great health care would be to become savvy enough to choose the right super-subspecialist for each health challenge you face. From a problem-oriented perspective, that would make complete and total sense.

However, studies have consistently shown, and shown conclusively, that the best health outcomes and lowest health care costs occur in places - countries, states, counties - where people have the greatest access to primary care. And the most effective health care systems in the world (e.g., Australia, Canada, England, and the Netherlands) have an equal number of primary care doctors and subspecialists doctors. By comparison, in the United States, fewer than one-third of physicians are trained in primary care.

The Institute of Medicine - now the National Academy of Medicine (NAM) - has defined primary care as, "the provision of integrated, accessible health care services by clinicians that are responsible for addressing a large majority of personal health care needs, developing a sustained partnership with patients, and practicing within the context of family and community." Based upon that definition, primary care is the only medical field defined by its processes rather than by a set of diseases.

Primary care physicians can be trained and certified in one (or more) of three specialties: Family Medicine, General Internal Medicine, and Pediatrics. Despite the fact that many young women only see a gynecologist, and residency programs in Obstetrics and Gynecology do include some training in primary care, OB/GYNs are generally not considered to be primary care physicians.

Why is primary care so important? It has to do with both the processes that characterize primary care and the kinds of people who choose to do it.

The Attributes of Primary Care

Based upon the NAM definition, primary care is characterized by eight attributes: accessibility, coordination, sustained care, comprehensiveness, partnership with patients, person-centeredness, integration, and accountability. Primary care physicians are expected to be experts in the application of these attributes just as a neurologist is an expert in diseases of the nervous system. Some attributes are organizational in nature (e.g., accessibility, coordination, and sustained care) while others are clinical or interpersonal (e.g. comprehensiveness, partnership, and person-centeredness). Integration and accountability apply to both categories.

The complexities involved in both the organizational and clinical aspects of primary care mean that a team approach is crucial. Most primary care practices therefore include an office manager, receptionists, billing staff, and medical assistants or nurses. Many also include nurse practitioners, physician assistants, and mental health professionals.

A relatively new type of practice called a "community health center" has evolved over the last 10 - 20 years. These federally-certified and supported practices, designed to preferentially care for medically underserved populations, but available to anyone, are required to include additional team members (e.g., social workers, pharmacists, and dentists).

Coordination, Advocacy, and Safety

Because the health care system is complex, and potentially dangerous, it can be extremely helpful to have an advocate within the system who knows and cares about you and has access to all of your health information. Coordination of care, under the supervision of an excellent primary care physician, can result in fewer unnecessary tests, fewer medication side effects and interactions, and fewer encounters with the health care system.

Bob Jamison was in his early 60s when I became his primary care physician. He was seeing a cardiologist for coronary artery disease and heart failure, a nephrologist for kidney disease and high blood pressure, an endocrinologist for Type 2 diabetes, and an ophthalmologist for diabetic eye care. He had also been to the emergency room on multiple occasions for attacks of gout, episodes of low blood sugar, and swelling with skin breakdown on his lower legs. He was taking 10 different prescription medications and was supposed to be following a low salt diabetic diet.

As I got to know Bob, I learned that his greatest joy in life was fishing. He owned a cabin on a nearby lake and a fishing boat and was known by his friends as "Bobber." However, fishing had become more difficult because of his gout, which had caused both pain and deformities of his finger joints. An emergency room doctor had recently started Bob on a gout medicine, which he had stopped along with most of his other medications when he developed a rash over his entire body. His lower legs had also become red and swollen up to his knees, and fluid was oozing through his skin in several places.

At our first visit I was able to help Bob identify the cause of his rash (a reaction to the new gout medicine) and to get him back on the most important of his medicines. Subsequently we were able to go over his entire health history and, in collaboration with his subspecialists, to make adjustments to his daily habits and medications that were compatible with his activities, especially fishing. He was able to reduce his total number of medicines by using alternative strategies to manage some symptoms. A different gout medicine and avoidance of certain foods reduced his joint pain and the swelling in his fingers, and adjustment of his diuretic (along with periodic leg elevation) dramatically reduced the swelling and redness in his legs, making fishing much more enjoyable.

Bob's important health care records are now in one place. They include consultation and emergency department notes, all of his test results, his advance directives, and his complete medical history and examination results. It is now possible to look across time and see what effect starting or stopping particular medications have had on his blood pressure, weight, and swelling.

Coordination of care and an advocate within the health care system are most important for people who need the health care system the most (e.g., older people with multiple health problems and children with multiple disabilities). However, because any of us could be in that situation at any point in time as a result of an accident or catastrophic health event, we should all establish a relationship with a primary care physician.

Comprehensiveness, Referrals, and Consultations

Primary care physicians are trained to help patients with 90% of their health-related needs. In fact, primary care physicians are not only able to help you with most of your health challenges, they are the experts in management of those conditions. Because common conditions are common, primary care physicians deal with them more often than subspecialists do and know better how to manage them.

When you do see a subspecialist, the expectation is that you will receive a specific diagnosis and definitive treatment. The buck stops there; they are the expert. This puts a great deal of pressure on subspecialists to "get it right." That pressure can result in excessive testing and treatment. "Errors of commission" — doing things that are excessive and unnecessary — are just as serious as errors of omission — doing too little.

Primary care doctors are under less pressure, particularly if a trusting doctor-patient relationship exists. They are therefore more comfortable suggesting watching and waiting when there is no immediate need to act. Studies have shown that, for a variety of common conditions, compared to subspecialists, family doctors generally arrive at the same conclusions, prescribe the same treatments when indicated, but order far fewer tests, and their patients do just as well.

Who Becomes a Primary Care Doctor?

As discussed in an earlier chapter, many students who make it through medical school incur substantial debt. Despite earning a salary for three years during residency training, half of the graduates of Family Medicine residencies still owe $150,000 or more. Because the salaries of primary care physicians are lower than those of most subspecialists, students who choose a career in primary care despite the financial disincentive are likely to do so because they enjoy the personal aspects of care.

In the 1970s, a study was done in which medical school graduates were asked what they would have done if they had not been admitted to medical school. A majority of future family physicians said they would have become teachers, counselors, or social workers, while physicians who had chosen a subspecialty were more likely to say they would have been scientists or engineers.

Several other studies have shown that the factors that predict whether a medical student will choose a career in primary care include: 1) being born and raised in a rural environment; 2) being a female; 3) being married; 4) having parents who are teachers or farmers; 5) having an interest in serving under-served or minority populations; and 6) a natural orientation to the emotional aspects of care.

Primary care is fundamentally relationship-based, and it involves care across the entire lifespan. For that reason it would be the most essential component of a goal-directed health care system. The role of your primary care doctor would be to know you well enough and understand the health care system well enough to help you decide whether problem-solving was the best strategy, whether you should see a subspecialist and, if so, which one.

How to Find a Good Primary Care Physician

Choosing a primary care doctor can be hard despite the increasing availability of the Internet. First, you will want to make a list of doctors who are covered under your health insurance plan. That list should be available from your insurance company. Then gather as much information as possible about the physicians on the list. You should be able to eliminate some based upon location, age range of patients seen, etc. Eliminate physicians who are not board certified in at least one of the three primary care specialties (Family Medicine, Internal Medicine, or Pediatrics). Then you will have to make some phone calls, since the online information is not always accurate and up-to-date.

You will want to be sure that the physician's *main* focus is primary care, not urgent care, hospital care, long term care, or a subspecialty like cardiology, endocrinology, gastroenterology, neurology, etc. While many primary care doctors, particularly those practicing in larger communities, no longer take care of patients in the hospital, you will probably want to know whether they do, and to which hospitals they usually send patients.

When choosing a primary care physician, remember that the hope is that you will be seeing this doctor for many years to come. Consider their age and plans for retirement. Take into consideration patient ratings, but recognize that a good bedside manner isn't always accompanied by up-to-date knowledge of medicine or good decision-making. Some of the worst doctors I have known get very high ratings from their patients. If the number of raters is low, remember that dissatisfied patients are probably more likely to take the time to provide ratings.

A more objective measure of competence is the doctor's history of sanctions (e.g., loss of hospital privileges, medical license, prescribing privileges, etc.). A helpful place to find this information is *http://www.docinfo.org/#/search/query*. If you find any significant sanctions, that should be a major red flag. Malpractice lawsuits filed against a doctor could also be important, but, unfortunately, there is no easy way to get that information at present.

Advice from your friends and family may be of some help in choosing a primary care physician, but again, people can be fooled by a doctor with a great personality. It is more helpful to get a recommendation from a health care professional. What you would hope to hear is that they would trust that doctor to care for members of their own family.

Doctors working at a university are more likely to be up-to-date medically and can often spend more time with you because their income is not totally dependent upon seeing patients, but they tend to have limited office hours, and you will probably be asked to allow students and residents to participate in your care. On the other end of the accessibility spectrum, a new model of primary care is emerging called "direct primary care." In these practices, for a monthly fee, you can have 24-7 access and more time during visits with your primary care doctor.

Personally, I would try to find a primary care physician who accepts Medicare and Medicaid patients even if you have neither. A willingness to care for patients who are often more challenging medically and for whom reimbursement rates are often lower suggests a concern for people over profit.

Nurse Practitioners and Physician Assistants

Nurse practitioners (NPs) are first trained as nurses, then as primary care clinicians, which gives them a unique perspective on health and healthcare. Their skills and perspective tend to be complementary to those of their physician supervisors. Because of the shortage of primary care physicians, NPs are becoming the main providers of primary care in many rural areas, often within community health centers.

Physician assistants (PAs) are trained and certified by physicians. They are somewhat less likely to choose to function independently, preferring to work side by side with and simply expanding the reach of their supervising physicians.

Both NPs and PAs increase access to primary care, which is a very good thing. Because their salaries are lower than those of physicians, they may be able to spend more time with you at each visit. They are well-trained to help you with simple challenges or for follow-up of a relatively stable chronic health condition.

NPs in particular may take a greater interest in prevention and on the impact of health challenges on quality of life. However, there are some disadvantages to having a NP or PA as your main primary care provider even though they are required to have a physician supervisor.

Because they have had less training than a doctor, NPs and PAs can help you with a somewhat smaller proportion of your health challenges. That means they may need to send you to a subspecialist sooner, subjecting you to the risk of over-testing and over-treatment. In addition, because of their somewhat lower stature within the medical hierarchy, they may have less influence over the course of events once you are referred to a subspecialist or admitted to a hospital. For example, if a surgeon recommends a questionable operation or a hospital-based physician recommends a premature discharge, an NP or PA may be less able to prevent that operation or that discharge from going forward.

In a goal-directed model, there is another theoretical disadvantage of getting most of your care from an NP or PA, and that is that goal-setting requires extensive knowledge of what is possible. NPs and PAs, because they have had less training, have less of that sort of knowledge. The experience acquired by primary care doctors during medical school and residency provides better preparation for this role.

The Importance of the Primary Care Doctor-Patient Relationship

Developing an ongoing, trusting relationship with a primary care doctor is incredibly important. Some would argue that it is the single most important thing you can do to improve the health care you receive. We all, from time to time, need someone outside of our circle of family and friends to talk to about sensitive or frightening things. And we want that person to know and care about us and have the knowledge and skills to help us face life's challenges.

However, relationship-building requires face time, and earlier in this book I suggested that you limit your number of encounters with the health care system. What is the appropriate middle ground?

Traditional annual physical examinations and lab tests are probably not the best use of time spent with your primary care doctor. However, I do recommend that everyone over the age of two see a primary care physician at least once a year to discuss personal health goals and develop or review an overall wellness plan. If during these wellness visits you have difficulty getting your physician to pay attention to your goals or to develop a personalized wellness plan, or if the doctor wants to perform tests and can't explain how they relate to your goals or plan, change doctors.

Many times you will be tempted to go directly to a subspecialist for a specific health concern. Sometimes that is the right thing to do, but before you decide to do that, consider the following points in favor of seeing or contacting your primary care physician first. Since primary care physicians are the experts at helping you manage 90% of health challenges, there's a pretty good chance you will get better care at a lower cost by seeing your primary care physician. If you do need to see a subspecialist, your primary care physician is more likely than you are to know which type of subspecialist you need and which subspecialist will provide the best care, given your particular circumstances. In addition, there's a greater likelihood that whatever happens, a record will end up in your primary care medical record if your primary care physician is involved in the process. Finally, the more opportunities you have for building a relationship with your primary care physician the better.

Another way to foster a relationship with your primary care physician is for multiple family members to see the same physician. That multiplies the opportunities for your doctor to get to know something about you as a person within your family context. For families with children, that can be accomplished by choosing a family doctor that takes care of children as well as adults. If there are no family doctors who see children or who meet your other criteria, you might have to take the children to a pediatrician, while the adults would need to see a family doctor or a general internist. There are also some physicians who have chosen to specialize in both Pediatrics and Internal Medicine.

Relationships depend upon both opportunity and compatibility. Some excellent primary care physicians will simply not be right for you or your family. One of the best family physicians I know is very directive in his approach. For example, he sometimes tells smokers not come to see him until they stop smoking since any other suggestions he might make would have little impact when compared to smoking cessation. Some people respond well to his style and some don't.

Other physicians I know feel very strongly that religion and spirituality should be a part of routine health care.

Goal-directed care requires a true partnership between you and your primary care doctor. That means that you need to have a certain level of knowledge about and comfort with each other. Both of you need to feel comfortable openly discussing disagreements and being honest about the direction you see things going for you. If that isn't possible, find a new doctor.

Other Red Flags

Many patients and primary care physicians are concerned that electronic medical records are interfering with the doctor-patient interactions essential to relationship building. Some physicians have hired "scribes" who handle the documentation requirements, leaving the physician free to communicate directly with patients. Others wait until after the visit to record their notes, while others involve their patients in the documentation process. If your physician seems more interested in the computer than in you, find another doctor.

The best way to generate income in primary care is to see more patients. That can be accomplished by spending less time listening and teaching, by scheduling more unnecessary follow-up visits, and by referring patients with anything complicated or time consuming to subspecialists. If your primary care physician sees more than 4 or 5 patients per hour, schedules routine follow-up visits more often than every 3 months even though your condition is stable, or seems unwilling to take the time to listen, switch doctors.

During medical school I spent several months working with a family physician in a small town in Wyoming. Prior to his arrival, the town had had two doctors who happened to be brothers. To hear people rave about those two doctors, you would have thought they deserved sainthood. Nearly everyone I met had been hospitalized for 6 weeks for rheumatic fever, an unusual complication of strep throat, and most of them said they owed their lives to one of the brothers. Another common report was that they had been told that if they had come in a day later the doctor might not have been able to save them. If a doctor says to you, "If you had come in a day later I might not have been able to save you," consider it a small red flag. Even if the statement is true, there is usually no reason to say it other than to elevate the doctor's importance.

Despite all of the progress made in medical science, your primary care physician will often be unable to give you a definitive answer to all of your questions. If your physician *never* says, "I don't know," consider that a red flag. You should also consider the following to be potential red flags: no after hours or weekend office hours, lack of phone availability after hours or direct referrals of after-hours calls to an emergency room, no back-up coverage when out of town, lack of office cleanliness, and poorly trained office staff.

Get Mostly Primary Care

1. Find and establish a long term relationship with a primary care physician.

2. If possible, encourage all of your family members to see the same primary care physician.

3. See your primary care physician for a wellness visit once a year.

4. In nearly all situations, consult your primary care physician first before seeing a subspecialist.

CHAPTER 14:

Getting Good Health Care

"I fear we are developing a group of competent technicians, treating disease, but not treating the whole patient. All medicine is judgment. I can bring anybody off the street and teach them how to cut and sew in three months. It is knowing when to operate and when not to operate that matters."

—Alton Ochsner

"The important question isn't how to keep bad doctors from harming patients; it's how to keep good doctors from harming patients."

—Atul Gawande

Good health care is health care that helps you achieve your goals. Bad health care is either not helpful (unnecessary, misdirected, or counterproductive) or harmful. Limiting your contacts with the health care system and cultivating a relationship with a good primary care physician will help you to get better health care, but there is more that you will need to do.

Goal-Directed Care

A significant proportion of the care provided by our current health care system is not helpful. However, it is possible for you to get mostly good health care. You already know that the knowledge and technical skills within the health care system are vast and powerful. The challenge is to access and apply that knowledge and those skills, only when necessary, to help you to achieve your personal health goals.

Before *every* encounter with the health care system—whether it is for a routine checkup or a new, potentially serious challenge—it is important that you prepare by reminding yourself about your health goals. This is absolutely critical since you will be entering a system with the power to overwhelm and redirect your thinking.

Length of Life

In previous chapters I have discussed the importance of prevention, and particularly primary (nutrition, physical activity, sleep, immunizations, seat belts, etc.) and secondary preventive measures (screening for cancer, heart attack risk, etc.). In most cases, you and your doctor will be in agreement about the value of those strategies. You are more likely to have trouble negotiating a goal-directed plan of care when you face potentially serious health challenges.

If you think you may be facing life or death decisions, the first question to ask yourself is whether staying alive is still a goal for you, and if not, why not? (Usually the answer will be yes, but it is still important to consider the question because the health care system is obligated to try to save your life until you tell them to stop.

When I was a junior in college, I remember thinking, and even stating out loud, that it would be perfectly okay if I died that day since I had had such a wonderful life. I was not depressed. In fact, I was gloriously happy. Then one night, walking home from a movie, my roommate and I were confronted by a small group of men with guns and chains. My roommate was beaten badly. A gun was pointed at my forehead. Just prior to being hit with the gun butt and knocked unconscious, I remember thinking how very much I did *not* want to die.

The best way to figure out whether staying alive is still a goal for you is to consider whether your current situation is actually worse than death and whether or not it is likely to improve. Worse than death means that you wouldn't want to be given antibiotics for a serious infection, you wouldn't want surgery for appendicitis, and you wouldn't want a blood transfusion if you were bleeding to death. In other words, you would welcome death as a better alternative than continuing to live.

If preventing premature death and disability is still a goal, then good health care (at any age) should include an assessment of your risk factors and advice about recommended preventive services.

As you age and begin to acquire treatable risk factors and health challenges (e.g., hypertension, diabetes, arthritis, osteoporosis, restless legs, etc.), much of the time you spend with your primary care doctor will be focused on treatment or management of those conditions. In order to keep the discussion focused on your goals, you will need to figure out which suggested strategies are intended to prolong your life, and which are intended to improve your quality of life. Then you can ask goal-relevant questions like: "By how much will this treatment increase my life expectancy or, for example, improve my endurance so that I can walk my dog? Your primary care doctor may have trouble answering those kinds of questions, but it still important to ask them.

In preparation for health care encounters, consider doing some homework. Even though it could be somewhat unsettling, you might want to begin by finding out what your average life expectancy is given your age, gender, and race/ethnicity. A good place to get that information is at *www. socialsecurity.gov/OACT/population/longevity.html*. You might also want to use the following life expectancy calculator developed in Canada, which takes into account lifestyle: *https:// www.projectbiglife.ca/life*. If you already have a potentially life-shortening health challenge like congestive heart failure or chronic lung disease, you could search for information on life expectancy – usually referred to as "prognosis" – for people with that condition.

One reason to know your life expectancy is that the effectiveness of preventive measures depends upon your living long enough to benefit. For example, you would need to stay alive for at least 10 years to benefit significantly from a colonoscopy or a prostate specific antigen test. And you would probably need to live at least 7 more years to benefit from a mammogram or pap test.

The United States Preventive Services Task Force (USPSTF) evaluates the effectiveness of primary and secondary preventive services. They have developed a free "app" that lists preventive services, with recommendations based on age and gender, or you can get this information directly from their website: *http://www.ahrq.gov/patients-consumers/index.html*. The USPSTF also provides the logic behind its recommendations including the average size of the benefits and risks.

As you conduct your research, be wary of information produced by organizations that stand to benefit from their own recommendations, or that might be otherwise biased by their commitments to their constituents. For example, onchologists (doctors who treat people with cancer) and the American Cancer Society may not always be the best sources of information on cancer screening.

Unfortunately, many screening tests have not been evaluated by the USPSTF. A few years ago, when I was 44 years old, I had surgery to remove a fistula tract, which is an abnormal connection between the rectum and the skin surface. Prior to the procedure, the surgeon wanted me to have a barium enema to see if I had Crohn's Disease, an inflammatory condition involving the intestine. He reminded me that people with Crohn's Disease are more likely to develop fistulas like mine. However, screening for Crohn's Disease in patients with fistulas has not been evaluated by the USPSTF.

I refused the test, arguing that diagnosing Crohn's Disease prior to having any symptoms (diarrhea and abdominal pain) would probably not prevent premature death or disability. Knowing that I had Crohn's Disease would only have made me, my family, the surgeon, and my primary care doctor worry. Treatment would probably not be recommended until I had symptoms. The surgeon argued that, if I had Crohn's, his repair might not heal well. I agreed to take that risk, and he grudgingly proceeded.

If the purpose of a health care visit is to seek help with a specific health challenge (e.g., swelling of your ankles), try to determine whether that condition could impact your survival or cause a future disability. In some cases the answer will be obvious. Significant damage to a vital organ like the heart will usually reduce life expectancy. In other cases, it may be less clear.

If it isn't that clear, ask your doctor, "Could this condition shorten my life or result in disability?" If the answer is "yes," then all decisions about further testing and treatment should be based upon estimates of their impact on your life (age at which you are likely to die) and health expectancies (age at which you would likely become completely disabled). The questions to ask are: "If I do what you are suggesting, how much longer could I expect to live (on average)? By how much would this treatment reduce my chance of future disability?" (After all, you wouldn't make a financial investment without knowing the average rate of return.)

In fact, doctors rarely discuss life expectancy with their patients, even though it often has profound implications on the decisions that must be made. When doctors are forced to estimate life expectancy, usually in patients with a terminal illness, studies have shown that they tend to be overly optimistic.

Some years ago, I took care of a 52-year-old man who had a heart that was barely strong enough to keep him alive, the consequence of years of alcohol and cocaine abuse. I told him that I didn't think he would live much longer without a heart transplant, and that to get on the transplant list he would have to give up alcohol and cocaine for at least 6 months. His response was, "That's OK doc, I never figured I would live beyond about 75." When I advised him that his projected life expectancy was less than 2 years without a transplant, he said, "Oh, so this is serious."

If you reach a point where survival is no longer a goal for you, tell your doctor. This can be a difficult conversation, of course, but it is a highly important step toward your goal of living out the rest of your life in the best possible manner. If any of your current medications are intended to prolong your life (e.g. blood pressure medicines), stop taking them. Find out what steps you need to take to make sure that no one tries to resuscitate you. If you don't want to be taken to a hospital, find out how to keep that from happening – if, for example, you are found confused on the floor by a neighbor or postal worker.

Quality of Life

Good health care is care that helps you maintain or increase your ability to do those things that make life worth living.

In many cases that involves diagnosing and treating specific abnormalities. However, unless you make your quality of life goals clear, problem-oriented care is likely to miss the mark for at least two reasons.

First, advances in testing methods have dramatically increased the number of abnormalities that can be detected. Most of these abnormalities will have no relevance at all to your personal health goals. However, once discovered, it is hard to ignore them. One test leads to another, and before you know it you are hopelessly caught up in a cascade of misguided tests and interventions. The best—and possibly only—way to prevent that from happening is to keep your goals clearly in mind, ask lots of questions, refuse tests that seem unrelated to your goals, and yell "Stop!" when you can see that things are going off course.

Second, the measures used by doctors to evaluate the effectiveness of treatments are symptoms, physical findings, and test results. Studies have shown that these measures don't always correlate with how well their patients are able to function. For example, in patients with rheumatoid arthritis, researchers found that there was almost no correlation between the number of inflamed joints or blood test results and patients' ability to participate in desired activities.

That doesn't mean that disease control isn't important; it is just not always sufficient for goal-achievement. You may also need rehabilitative therapies, adaptive equipment, vocational training, and/or mental health support, for example. It is much more likely that treatment for specific diseases will help you achieve your goals if you are very clear with your doctors about what your goals are.

So, when considering your quality of life goals, here are some crucial questions to consider:

During a typical day, what are the things that you wish you could do better, and what is keeping you from doing them as well as you would like to?

What are your passions, the things that make life worthwhile for you, which give life meaning and purpose?

What would you like to be able to do that you can't do now?

Other Aspects of Good Care

Good care should, whenever possible, be evidence-based. That is, there should be reliable evidence that what you decide to do might actually work.

Fortunately, there is an ever-increasing amount of reliable information on the Internet to help you determine which treatments and tests are well supported by research. I recommend starting with the following sites: *http://www. cochrane.org/*, *https://nccih.nih.gov/health/atoz.htm*, and *http:// familydoctor.org*. Good sites pertaining to children's' health issues are *https://www.healthychildren.org* and *http://www. aboutkidshealth.ca*.

Unfortunately, we live in a world in which preying on people's fears and misfortunes can be both financially rewarding and low risk. It can be difficult to know when someone is trying to sell you snake oil. A great site to go to for information about treatments that seem too good to be true is *http://www.quackwatch.com*.

Good care should also include discussions and documentation of values and preferences, including advance directives regarding end of life care, as previously discussed. And good health care should be characterized by generous amounts of support, reassurance, education, and encouragement and referral to additional sources of information.

Putting it all Together

As I am writing this book I am 68 years old. I still enjoy life a great deal. Given my personal risk factors, I can expect to live to be around 84 on average. Because of my risk factors (elevated cholesterol and blood pressure, and a family history of heart attacks), I am most likely to die from a heart attack or stroke. The strategies most likely to extend my life are moderate physical activity, a diet rich in vegetables, fruits, nuts, whole grains, and olive oil, taking a blood pressure medicine called an ACE inhibitor, taking 81mg of aspirin once a day, and taking a cholesterol lowering medicine called a statin, all of which I am doing. I don't need to have my cholesterol level checked regularly, because I am already doing what I can to lower it. Annual flu shots make sense since they are easy and low risk. I am up to date on pneumonia, shingles, and tetanus vaccinations – also easy. I had a colonoscopy two years ago because colon cancer is fairly easy to prevent by removing polyps. I would have enormous regrets if a I died of colon cancer and had done nothing to prevent it.

While there are many activities that I enjoy, I particularly like thinking and writing. And since these activities are so important to me, I am careful to avoid damaging my brain. I don't drink excessive amounts of alcohol, and I don't do things that are likely to result in a head injury like driving a motorcycle, jumping out of airplanes, or diving off of cliffs. In retirement, I keep my brain engaged by writing, reading, engaging in social activities, taking classes, and maintaining contact with former academic colleagues through contract work. I also enjoy physical activities like basketball, hiking, yard work, and gardening. Since I have a tendency to develop episodes of low back pain, I do exercises to strengthen my back and abdominal muscles, and I am careful when lifting or twisting. Now that I have two very young grandsons being able to bend and lift have become even more important.

When my wife and I recently moved from Oklahoma to North Carolina, I downloaded the advance directive documents for my new home state from *http://www.caringinfo. org/i4a/pages/index.cfm?pageid=3289*, completed them, and have asked that they be scanned into my medical record. Since the same record is used in the hospital I would use, they should be accessible there as well. I have established a relationship with a primary care doctor, and he knows these things about me though I have only seen him twice. His understanding of me as a person is enhanced because he also takes care of my wife.

I hope my story gives you hope that it is possible get goal-directed health care from our problem-oriented health care system. But, remember, I have several advantages. I have been trained in clinical medicine, I know how physicians think, and I understand how the system works. I have also been thinking about goal-directed care for a long time. For you to be as successful, you will need to know the kinds of questions to ask, when to ask them, and when and how to graciously decline your doctors' advice when it doesn't serve your needs. In the next chapter, I will provide some examples of how to do those things.

Make Sure the Care You Receive
Relates to Your Goals

1. In preparation for every visit to a health care professional, remind yourself of your personal health goals.

2. Try to determine whether and how much the health care interventions being suggested are likely to impact your goals.

3. Learn as much as you can about your personal risk factors for premature death and disability and what to do about them. Find or calculate your estimated life expectancy if possible.

4. Make sure you tell health care professionals what you need and want to do and how your health conditions seem to be impacting your ability to do them. Ask how each health care recommendation is likely to affect your ability to do those things that make life meaningful and enjoyable.

5. Make sure you have completed and given family members and health care providers copies of your advance directives and told them the conditions under which you would not want to be kept alive.

CHAPTER 15:

Nuts, Bolts, Techniques, and Scripts

"Today you are You, that is truer than true. There is no one alive who is Youer than You."

—*Dr. Seuss*

In this book, I have focused primarily on concepts, providing specific examples to help you to understand them. In this chapter, I will suggest some simple, practical steps that you can take with your personal physician to make sure you get the type of goal-directed care I've been discussing.

It is possible for you to view health and health care through a different lens (goal-directed vs. problem-oriented) without jeopardizing your relationship with your doctor, but it will require some knowledge, techniques (strategies), and scripts (ways of saying things). Your health care providers want you to do well. If you are patient and respectful, you can get the assistance that you need, even from a problem-oriented system.

The main weakness of the problem-oriented medical model is that it focuses attention on abnormalities rather than on you as a person. To get your needs met, you will have to keep bringing the focus back to you and your particular needs and circumstances. When you do that, your doctors may become a little uncomfortable, even anxious. There are three reasons for that discomfort:

They are used to discussing your medical problems and their treatment. All of their techniques and scripts are problem-oriented. When you shift the focus, they will be taken out of their comfort zone.

They also won't know the answers to some of your very appropriate questions, and they may think you are questioning their competence.

They may assume that bringing your personal goals into the conversation will take more time and energy that they don't have.

Keeping that in mind, here are some ways to help your doctor help you.

---

1. When speaking with your doctor, keep bringing the discussion back to the things that matter to you (i.e., your goals) by asking goal-oriented questions.

Let's say you have gone to your primary care doctor for a preventive care visit. The conversation might go something like this.

You: I'm doing very well right now, enjoying retirement and especially the grandkids. I came in today to find out what I can do to stay alive as long as possible (as long as I am still enjoying life).

Your Doctor: That's great! I'm so glad to hear that. For a person of your age and gender, we recommend that you have the following immunizations and screening tests.

You: OK. That sounds easy enough. Remember; I'm 70 years old. Given my life expectancy, do you think I will still benefit from those tests?

Your Doctor: Great question. Yes, I think so.

You: OK. Go ahead and order them for me. Now, knowing what you know about me, what do you think I'm most likely to die from? Is there anything else that I can do to reduce my risk of dying from those things?

Your Doctor: Another good question. Based upon the risk factors that I know about, including your family history, I'd say you are most likely to die from cancer. We will be screening you for some types of cancers, but perhaps it would also be a good idea for you to have a thorough skin exam and to learn to check your thyroid, testicles, and lymph nodes regularly. You should also learn the warning signs of cancer. I think I have a handout on those.

You: I also want to make sure that you have my advance directives in your record. Can you check to be sure that you have both my living will and my durable power of attorney for health care? Will that information automatically be sent to the hospital if I have to be hospitalized for some reason, or should I take copies to them as well? And if there is a place to put it in your record, I also want you to indicate that I would not want to be kept alive if I can no longer recognize members of my own family.

II. If you are seeing your doctor because you have a new symptom, such as lower back pain, your interaction with the doctor might go something like this.

You: I have a fairly constant pain in my lower back. It's making it difficult for me to sit for very long, and that makes it hard for me to do my work since I have a desk job. I also can't play basketball, which is my main source of exercise.

Your Doctor: Well, based upon what you've told me, my examination, and taking into account your age and overall health, I think you've probably

injured one of the discs in your lumbar spine –
your lower back. The pain should get better in a
few weeks. I will give you a prescription for something to relieve the pain. If it doesn't get better, or
if you experience persistent numbness or weakness
or trouble with your bowels or bladder, we might
have to do some blood tests, back X-rays, and
possibly an MRI scan.

You: That makes sense. Do you have time for a few
more questions?

Your Doctor: Sure.

You: Why did this happen? Was it something I did
(that I shouldn't do again)?

Your Doctor: Disk injuries are really common. If you
can't remember a specific injury event, it will be
hard to figure out exactly when it happened. You
might have had it for years and it is just now
beginning to cause you trouble.

You: As you may recall, I'm an architect. I have to do a
fair amount of sitting both at work and at home.
Do you have any suggestions about what I should
do about work and other activities?

Your Doctor: The pain is likely to be worst when you
are sitting. If it is possible, you should either work

from a standing position or at least get up and walk around every few minutes. That could help. They make a type of seat that puts you in a kneeling position, which might work better than sitting.

You: Is this injury likely to happen again? If so, what can I do to try to prevent it?

Your Doctor: Great questions! Yes, I'm afraid that most people with this problem have intermittent episodes for the rest of their lives. I can refer you to a physical therapist who can teach you some techniques and give you some exercises that could reduce reoccurrences.

You: If it does happen again, is there something I can do so that I don't have to come back in to see you?

Your Doctor: As long as the symptoms are the same and you don't have any numbness or weakness in your legs or trouble controlling your bladder or bowels, you really shouldn't need to come in. I will give you a refill on the pain medication in case you need it. Unfortunately it will only last 6 months. However, if you call the office during regular office hours, I will tell my staff to refill it.

You: For future reference, would it help if I write down my questions and bring them with me to my visits with you?

> Your Doctor: I actually like it when my patients do
> that, as long as you realize we usually only have
> 15 minutes. If you are pretty sure the visit will last
> longer than that, tell my appointment secretary to
> give you back-to-back slots.

III. When considering what to do about your symptoms, your primary care doctor is thinking, "Is there an effective treatment available for this condition?" You will want your doctor to also consider whether treatment is necessary at that point in time? That is, will it benefit you enough to justify the risks?

Let's say you have a fever and a cough; you are coughing up yellow phlegm, and your doctor has diagnosed bronchitis.

> Your Doctor: You have bronchitis, a bacterial compli-
> cation of the cold you had last week. I'm going
> to prescribe an antibiotic that I want you to take
> three times a day for a week.

> You: I was planning to stay home from work tomor-
> row and Friday and the weekend. How long is
> this infection likely to last if I just stay at home
> and rest? Is there any danger in not taking the
> antibiotic?

> Your Doctor: No…probably no real danger. I guess
> it could progress to pneumonia, but if you want
> to try rest and fluids for a few more days, and if

you promise to call me if you are getting worse… more short of breath, more chest pain, higher fever, etc… I'm OK with waiting on the antibiotics. In fact, since the weekend is coming up, why don't I give you a prescription for the antibiotic, which you can fill if you get worse, or tear up if you get better? Feel free to call if you aren't sure what to do.

IV. When you have a chronic health challenge, try to find out whether the treatment recommendations are intended to increase your length of your life or to improve your current or future quality of life.

Let's say you have developed lupus, a condition in which your body's natural defense system is attacking your own cells and organs.

<u>You</u>: If you have time, I have some questions.

<u>Your Doctor</u>: Of course.

<u>You</u>: Is lupus the type of condition that can shorten my life?

<u>Your Doctor</u>: Unfortunately, since lupus can affect different people in different ways, we don't have a perfect answer to that question. I can tell you that in the 1950s nearly 50% of lupus patients died within 5 years of their diagnosis. Now 80-90%

lupus patients have a normal lifespan. I can't say for sure how much of that improvement is due to advances in treatment, but certainly some of it is.

You: Will the treatments you are recommending only relieve my symptoms, or will they actually prolong my life or prevent future disability?

Your Doctor: Some, like the anti-inflammatory medicines, are primarily focused on improving your symptoms. The hydroxychloroquine (Plaquenil), on the other hand, has been shown to prevent organ damage and prolong life.

You: Now that I have lupus, what am I most likely to die from?

Your Doctor: The most common causes of death in people with lupus are heart attacks and strokes. Other causes include damage to other organs like the kidneys and infections related to both the disease and the medications we use to treat it on the body's natural defense mechanisms.

You: Besides Plaquenil, is there anything else that I can do to prolong my life?

Your Doctor: Consistently taking the Plaquenil is really important. It is also important for you and your primary care doctor to address any other risk factors you have for heart attacks and strokes. And you should definitely quit smoking. Smoking increases the risk of blood clots in people with lupus and it reduces the effectiveness of the Plaquenil. Smoking also increases your risk of developing pneumonia.

<u>You</u>: Could any of the treatments you are suggesting for my symptoms actually shorten my life?

<u>Your Doctor</u>: Yes. All medications can potentially cause harm. Medicines used to keep your defense mechanisms from damaging your organs can also increase your risk of infections and cancer. That's why you need to report new symptoms to your doctors sooner and get treated earlier than if you were not taking those medicines.

V. When your doctor suggests that you have some tests:

<u>Your Doctor</u>: I'd like to order a few more tests.

<u>You</u>: What sorts of things are you looking for?

<u>Your Doctor</u>: These tests will look for a number of abnormalities in your liver, kidneys, and blood that I might not be able to detect on examination. At this point, I'm not looking for anything specific. There are a number of tests in the panels I

am ordering. I would feel better knowing that you don't have something serious.

You: If you don't suspect something specific, I'd really rather not go looking for trouble. Is there any danger in waiting to see if my symptoms get worse?

Notes:

1. *As a general rule, you should not agree to have tests to make the doctor feel better.*

2. *You should be especially hesitant to agree to be tested for things that are unlikely. Since no test is perfectly accurate, false positive results are common when the condition you are being tested for is unlikely.*

Your Doctor: There is a blood test we can do to see if you could have cancer of your ovary.

You: What do you think the probability is that I have cancer in my ovary?

Your Doctor: Very low, especially considering the normal ultrasound. But it would make me feel better knowing that you don't have cancer.

You: Then I think I'll pass on the blood test. I'm

concerned that if the result is positive, it is likely
to be a false positive.

*Doctors sometimes order tests because of the fear of malpractice
lawsuits. You can prevent that from happening by agreeing to
take responsibility for the decision not to be tested. The doctor
will make a note to that effect in the record and feel reassured.*

---

*VI. When treatment or management is discussed, make sure that
you are actually able to do what is being suggested.*

Your Doctor: You will need to take this medicine twice
a day 30 minutes before breakfast and 30 minutes
before supper.

You: Will it matter if I don't eat breakfast? I almost
never do, and my supper schedule varies depending upon how late I have to work.

Your Doctor: Well, the medicine needs to be taken on
an empty stomach, so take one in the morning
shortly after you get up. What is the earliest you
ever eat supper?

You: Occasionally I eat at 5, but more often its 6 or 7.

Your Doctor: How about if you take the second dose
at 9PM. That should be long enough after supper.
Would that work?

VII. If you have a chronic condition that will require regular visits to your doctor over a period of years, discuss with your doctor what tests will need to be done, and how frequently (and, of course, the reasons for them). Once you have settled on a mutually agreeable plan, take responsibility yourself for making sure it is carried out.

Your Doctor: I want to see you again in a month.

You: What will happen at that visit?

Your Doctor: I just want to be sure your symptoms are improving and that the treatment is working as it should.

You: Is there anything you need to do, like an examination or tests, or could I just call and report my progress and symptoms to your nurse?

Your Doctor: I guess so. Yes, that should work. How about if you report in with my nurse at least once each month, and I'll see you again in the office in 3 months?

You: Will you want to see me at some sort of regular intervals? If so, I might be able to help make sure that happens and that I schedule any tests ahead of those visits so we will be able to discuss the results. Can we make a plan like that?

VIII. When you are seriously ill:

Your Doctor: For the type of cancer you have, we use three different medicines in combination with radiation therapy.

You: On average, how long do people like me, with my type of cancer, live without treatment? And how long, on average, can I expect to live with the treatment you're suggesting? (I realize you can only provide averages, but I would still find the information helpful.)

Your Doctor: On average people with your type of cancer can expect to live about one year without treatment, but it varies a lot. With treatment, it depends upon how well your cancer responds to the treatment.

You: I understand, but can you tell me the average results? How likely is it that my cancer will respond? If it does, how likely is it that the cancer will be gone for good? And I want to read up on my cancer on the computer when I get home. Can you write down the specific name and extent of my cancer and the medicines you are planning use, so that I can find the correct information?

IX. *Make it OK for the doctor to say, "I don't know"*

> You: You may not know the answer to this question, and it's OK if you don't, but what are the chances that my aneurysm will burst during my lifetime, or in the next 10 years?

or…

> You: This is a really tough question, I know. But given my current medical conditions, what do you think I am most likely to die from? Are there any ways, aside from the medicines you have prescribed, that I can reduce my risk of dying from those things?

X. Lastly, here are some things you can do to save the doctor and office staff time, so they will have more time to talk with you. Increasing documentation requirements have reduced the amount of time your doctor can spend with you, but you can relieve some of the administrative burden if you bring the following with you to doctor visits:

First Visit Only (or any visit when the information has changed):

1. A list of any allergies that you have to medicines, foods, and things that might contact your skin (e.g., latex). There is no need to list all of the things that cause you to have hay fever or nasal congestion.

2. A list, in chronological order, of all of the times you have been in the hospital and the reasons you were there.

3. A list of your grandparents, parents, brothers and sisters, and children. Beside each family member, list the health problems they have had and the date of their death if they are no longer alive.

4. Copies of your advance directives.

Every Visit:

1. All of the medicines you take on a regular basis, including over-the-counter medicines and supplements. Bring these medications with you *to every visit*. A typed list is nice but not as good as the actual pill containers with the pills in them.

2. If you are changing pharmacies, bring the name, address, and phone number of the new pharmacy.

3. A list of things you would like to get from the visit (for example):

    a. The doctor's opinion about what is causing the pain in my stomach

    b. Things I can do to relieve it

    c. An estimate of how long it is likely to last

    d. A note for work for the doctor to sign (if necessary)

CHAPTER 16:
Final Thoughts

Most of us are, by nature, goal-directed. The decisions we make generally relate to the outcomes we have in mind, and, for that reason, most service organizations and businesses have adopted a goal-directed approach. The hotel industry has learned that customer satisfaction is highest when their staff focuses on making each guest's experience the best it can be rather than on providing the same experience for all guests. Fast food restaurants design their products and packaging to be compatible with the conditions under which they are likely to be consumed (e.g. while driving). When you see an attorney, one of the first things she will want to know is your goal.

Perhaps the best example is the financial planning industry. When my wife and I visit with our financial planner, he asks a number of goal-oriented questions: How long do you expect to live based upon your current health and your risk factors? What do you want to be able to do before you die, and how much is that going to cost? Do you expect to inherit any money; if so, approximately when and how much? Do you anticipate any major expenses (college tuitions, weddings, relocations, etc.)? How much money would each of you need to live on if the other one dies first?

Imagine having that kind of frank conversation with your primary care physician.

As we have seen, the current health care system is designed to solve problems; and it is really good at it. Health care professionals, chosen for their aptitude in science, are trained to use scientific principles and techniques to prevent and treat human diseases. The implied assumption is that perfect health is defined by the absence of biological risk factors and malfunctions. Based upon that assumption, every person has the same health goal, to be biologically "normal." While that way of thinking has resulted in improvements in life expectancy and quality of life, it has also contributed to rising health care costs, and it has tended to dehumanize care.

The goal-directed approach to health and health care that I have suggested and discussed in this book would in no way discard or diminish the importance of scientific advances. It would simply provide a framework within which those advances and advances yet to come, could be applied more strategically, collaboratively, and humanely.

While there are indications that the goal-directed approach to health care might eventually emerge, the obstacles are substantial. Therefore, in the mean time, it will be up to you to wrestle goal-oriented care from a problem-oriented system. To do that you will need to:

1. Carefully consider your health-related goals.

2. Think about the factors that could put you at risk for premature death and disability. Discuss them with your doctor and decide what to do to address them.

3. Think about the activities, relationships, and passions that, for you, make life worth living. Consider things that you can do now to preserve or enhance your ability to continue to enjoy those things for as long as possible.

4. Periodically consider what conditions would, for you, be worse than death recognizing that your thoughts about this may change over time. Tell key people such as family members and your primary care doctor.

5. Understand and embrace your capacity as a human being to continue to grow and develop throughout life physically, emotionally, and spiritually. Learn to view obstacles as opportunities.

6. Accept the fact that death is inevitable. Think and talk with others about the values you feel strongly about as they pertain to death and dying. Complete and distribute advance directive documents. Make sure that potential decision-makers know your values and wishes.

7. Learn as much as you can — from reliable sources — about how your body works and the challenges that may affect your ability to achieve your goals.

8. Learn as much as you can about how the health care system works and how health care professionals are selected, trained, evaluated and paid. Do what you can to help your health care professionals help you by preparing for visits and providing them with the information they need.

9. Take good care of yourself so you don't have to seek health care very often.

10. Stay physically active, eat a healthy diet ("good food, not too much, mostly vegetables"), and get enough sleep;

11. Avoid tobacco products and abstain from or use alcohol in moderation;

12. Take care of your teeth;

13. Protect your skin, vision, and hearing;

14. Practice responsible sex;

15. Get recommended immunizations;

16. Recognize and try to reduce factors the put you, in particular, at risk for premature death and disability.

17. Because thinking is essential to nearly all meaningful human activities, get as much formal education as possible and then keep learning. Stay engaged in the activities you enjoy with people you enjoy being with.

18. Develop a long term relationship with a primary care physician.

19. Encourage all of your health care providers to consider your personal goals whenever you seek their advice and assistance.

20. When health challenges arise, learn all you can about them (do your homework).

21. Only agree to tests and treatments that have a reasonable chance of helping you achieve your health goals.

22. Be extremely cautious about taking medications, understand the purpose and potential hazards of each medication, and, if medications are essential, keep the total number of medicines you take to the absolute minimum necessary to support your goals.

23. Think about the trade-offs you are willing to make between your health-related goals.

24. When choosing between quality of life and length of life, remember that quality doesn't matter after you are dead, and that people tend adapt better to disabilities than they thought they would.

25. When choosing between quality of life and personal growth and development, remember that the latter tends to be what people value most in the end.

26. When choosing between life sustaining treatments and a good death, recognize that the health care system will usually err on the side of treatment. It will be up to you to find out all you can about the benefits and risks of the proposed treatment, consult with family members and other confidents, and then make the best decision you can.

Acknowledgements

While I have always enjoyed writing, this book would never have been written had it not been for the persistent encouragement of Dr. John Belzer. The idea of goal-directed health care first occurred to me around 1990, the year I hired John to help me run the University of Oklahoma Geriatric Education Center. John recognized long before I did that the most important audience for the idea was not going to be health care professionals but patients.

For nearly 25 years I gave lectures, facilitated case discussions, wrote journal articles, and promoted the idea to colleagues and medical audiences. Thankfully some, including Dr. Cheryl Aspy, Ms. Jacque Cook, Dr. Peter Winn, Dr. John Zubialde, and Dr. Dewey Scheid at the University of Oklahoma, and Dr. David Waters at the University of Virginia, Dr. Paul James at the State University of New York in Buffalo, and Dr. Bill Smucker at the Family Medicine Residency Program at Summa Health in Akron, Ohio provided reassurance when I needed it most. Dr. Zsolt Nagykaldi, outstanding researcher and the best computer programmer I have ever met, conceptualized and developed the goal-oriented registry mentioned in Chapter 9, which has been well-accepted and extremely helpful to patients who have used it, but which is unfortunately still underutilized by clinicians.

After banging heads with the health care establishment for years, I finally realized that John had been right all along. However, writing a book is hard work, and it is particularly hard for a physician to write a book for non-physicians. A basketball acquaintance told me about Jeremy Hawkins, a young novelist who took on editing jobs to make a living. His lack of knowledge about the health care system was just what I needed. I am also grateful to two long-time friends, Ken Ross and Lyndee Knox who read drafts of the book and made key suggestions, many of which I used to improve it.

The book would still not have been written absent the unconditional love and support of my wife, Sandy, and my mother, Nelda, my two most enthusiastic cheerleaders.

ABOUT THE AUTHOR

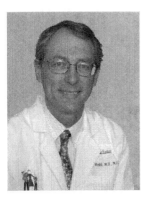

James W. Mold, MD, MPH

George Lynn Cross Emeritus Research Professor

Department of Family and Preventative Medicine

University of Oklahoma Health Sciences Center Oklahoma City, OK

Jim Mold is a George Lynn Cross Emeritus Professor of Family Medicine and a consultant to the University of Oklahoma Health Sciences Center. Educated at the University of Michigan and Duke Medical School and trained at the University of Rochester, he first worked as a physician in a remote village in West Africa, then in a small town in North Carolina, and finally as a faculty member at the University of Oklahoma, where he also practiced and taught geriatric medicine and conducted research in primary care practices. In 2008 he was elected to the National Academy of Medicine. While he has published more than 170 research articles and book chapters, this is his first book. Dr. Mold now lives in Chapel Hill, N.C. with his wife, Sandy, and their golden retriever, Lily.

For more information about goal-directed healthcare or to contact the author, go to: www.goaldirectedhealthcare.org.